MoveWell Secrets

MoveWell University, LLC
www.movewelluniversity.com
drtodd@movewellu.com
ISBN 13: 978-1-945028-16-8

This book is not intended as a substitute for the medical advice of physicians. The reader should regularly consult a physician in matters relating to his/her health and particularly with respect to any symptoms that may require diagnosis or medical attention.

MoveWell Secrets

TODD PICKMAN, DC

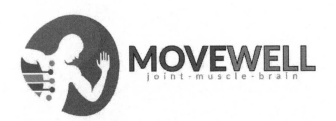

This book is dedicated to my superhero wife Linda for being so understanding and supportive as to why I had to work 15 hours a day for months on end to develop, refine and fine-tune the systems that inspired this book. Not to sound cliché, but I couldn't have done this without you in my corner, my ultimate supporter.

I love you and our beautiful Grayson (ands three original kiddos—the dogs).

Contents

Foreword

PRIOR TO BEING, "THE MOVEMENT BASED CHIRO-practor" I applied what I had learned in Chiropractic school when treating patients. For example, when a patient presented with a knee complaint I would administer as many orthopedic tests as I could think of to come up with a diagnosis and devise a treatment plan.

After four years into practice I was applying this same philosophy to an elite runner. This female runner had already been to the orthopedic surgeon, physical therapist and had MRI's and x-rays performed (all negative). Knee pain had prevented her from running for the past 3 months. If you treat athletes you know it takes quite the emotional and spiritual toll when they can't do the activities they love.

She said I was her last hope. About midway thru my initial consultation and performing a Clarke's Patellar Grind test, I stopped cold in my tracks. I just hung out there for a few minutes with her leg in my hands and me staring at her knee. When she asked, "Are you okay" I replied, "No. I am not okay".

I was doing all the same tests that the other clinicians had performed. I knew I wasn't as good as the orthopedic surgeon at these tests so what made me think performing the same tests would net a different result? I felt stupid and like I wasn't serving my patient well. I knew at that point I had to do something different to feel fulfilled in my practice.

I decided to stop looking simply for a diagnosis and rely more on assessing a person's movement and correcting faulty movement patterns. Getting people off of the table and evaluating how they move has made all the difference in my practice. About 14 years later I have read most, if not all, movement assessment books, scientific literature, taken courses, and earned numerous certifications. I have taken what I learned and applied in practice with phenomenal results.

What has taken me 14 years (and thousands of dollars and numerous mistakes) to learn has been consolidated into one resource. This book. Dr. Todd Pickman has not only laid out the rationale for a movement-based approach but delivers all of the other variables that nobody out there has organized into clear, step-by-step systems. You will benefit emotionally, spiritually, and financially by looking at the human body in the way both he and I feel is the right way. In motion.

I wish I had this resource many years ago. This book is the 'cheat sheet' to cover the wide array of variables that a chiropractor fails to consider in their quest to assess and improve human movement AND to make it work in practice. Both you and your patients will thank you for spending the time to read what Dr. Pickman has laid out.

—Edward C. Le Cara, DC, PhD, MBA, ATC, CSCS
Board Certified in Sports & Rehabilitation
www.TheMovementBasedChiropractor.com

CHAPTER 1

The Evolution of Exercise

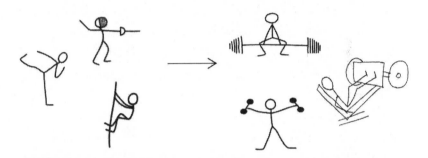

MY NAME IS DR. TODD PICKMAN. I'M A CHIROPRAC-
tor by trade and the owner of a clinic called Gonstead
Spine & Wellness, out here in Meridian, Idaho. As the
clinic director, I started this thing called MoveWell University, as an
idea awhile back, and I really couldn't have done it without Tony
Ammirati. He's had a background as a personal trainer for 15 years,
and he's been a team member in our clinic for some time now. His
background varies from kettlebells to martial arts, and he's primarily
focused on helping us continue this project called MoveWell University. Tony and I first started talking about functional movement
and applying it to the healthcare model. Since then, we started this
project called MoveWell Secrets, which is what this book is about.
But first, why should you care and why should you listen to me?

I've been in clinical practice since 2003, and I had the opportunity to always be around success ever since I graduated chiropractic
school; it's all that I know. I started off my first eight years in practice
in a very successful, multi-chiropractor clinic in Albuquerque, New
Mexico. I primarily practiced in a strict Gonstead, adjustment-only

model, until I began to venture out, looking for what else I could do for my patients to improve outcomes and further challenge my clinical expertise. I found curve-correction, the technique touted to be the most evidence-based, peer-reviewed, non-surgical spinal corrective care system in the world: Chiropractic BioPhysics.

My wife and I relocated to Eagle, Idaho, to partner in one of the biggest chiropractic clinics to open in the country, Ideal Spine Health Center. I realized, just shy of the first year into building a patient base in this clinic, that I had a different calling. My wife and I left to go open our own unique vision, Gonstead Spine & Wellness. We first worked out of a temporary space, while our clinic was being constructed, and we finally opened our doors on July 4, 2014. From that point forward, we grew quickly — very quickly. And not only did our patient numbers grow, but I had this burning desire to dial in my clinical approach, to improve my outcomes even more. But I knew I was still missing something, and that something was movement. I was measuring movement with my patients and I certainly wasn't addressing it. I didn't know where to begin, but I jumped in 1,000 percent, and three years later, we now have one of the most systematic, organized, results-based, reproducible systems in functional movement and corrective exercise.

I understand that our audience is varied. There are people who are reading this who fully understand functional movement. They know what it is and they're doing it themselves. They've been immersed in it. They already know the Functional Movement Screen (FMS) and Selective Functional Movement Assessment (SFMA). They've been to seminars, and they are reading this book to see if they can pick up any gems or things that we can share with them.

Then we have the other end of the spectrum, where some doctors do nothing with exercise, nothing with movement. They've heard about it, but it sounds too complicated and overwhelming. Some doctors may not exercise themselves, and so they're thinking, "Ok, this isn't my platform. It's not my arena." I would argue that understanding corrective exercise and functional movement NEEDS to be on the radar for ALL chiropractors who want to do the best job for their patients. This is one of the main things that I'm going to try to accomplish moving through the MoveWell Secrets.

We could have called this "The Five Main Secrets That You Need to Know About Exercise" or "Three Shortcuts for Implementing Functional Movement Into Your Practice," but we decided to keep it transparent and straightforward. No fluff, and no holds barred. In creating this book, we hoped to initially capture your attention with the anticipation that you will get a ton of value out of this read, so even though we didn't put some really sensationalized title on this whole thing, it's going to be awesome.

We're going to start with where we came from why this is even important, where we're at right now, and the future of MoveWell. Don't think of this program as an exercise methodology. This is true healthcare. It's health. It's longevity. If you are a healthcare professional, a health counselor or coach, or you guide people in health in any way, you need to know this stuff.

Let's get into it. So first off, let's discuss the evolution of exercise. Back in the day exercise gyms used to be what? They were gymnasiums. I have some old pictures of what gyms used to look like. They had climbing ropes, balance beams, fencing and gymnastics, and all that kind of stuff. And the world was really different. In the last four or five decades, the fitness industry has really changed a lot. Where did all of this thinking start and where has it evolved over the last few decades? The son of the founder of the chiropractic profession, BJ Palmer, had an interesting clinical approach. His clinic was indeed an exercise facility. If you saw pictures of his clinic, it was a full gymnasium. He'd be adjusting patients in one part of the building, while he had other patients climbing over obstacles and rolling or climbing ropes. His clinic had balance beams and gymnastic rings. I remember, when I originally first saw his clinic, I thought it was weird to incorporate all of that exercise stuff, especially in that fashion. I now realize I felt that way because I wasn't in this arena yet, and now I can see how appropriate this setup actually was. BJ Palmer was far ahead of his time. And now we've gone away from that, because places like that don't really exist anymore unless you're a gymnast.

On the topic of gymnastic rings, this used to be a common form of exercise back in the day. Ring work has fallen out of use by a lot of people because it is now viewed as being really advanced. Nowadays, when we're very sedentary and a lot of the population doesn't work-out at all, trying to get them up on rings is going to be nearly impossible. The nice thing about the methods and protocols we use is we can take anyone from a complete beginner who's never exercised to an advanced athlete, and we have things we can do with them. As we get through the chapters in this book, we will address this concept more, for sure.

The goal is to take someone who is dysfunctional, whether they are in pain or have no pain at all, and get them moving functionally and have them perform activities that carry over into their normal activities of daily living. But the goal with our patients, the light at the end of the tunnel (and this is how we communicate with our patients too), is to get them into some level of strength and power and fitness. It doesn't matter if they're 90 years old or if they're 9 years old. The first goal is to get them moving in a healthy way and then progressing them to some level of strength, power, and fitness.

When people start getting rid of these dysfunctions and begin to move better, they're going to want to move more. They are excited to enjoy this new range of movement that they may have been missing for years, decades, or even since they were a small child. From a doctor's perspective, at least in my mind, many doctors are a little intimidated to want to really talk about how their patients should be exercising. Almost like when a patient comes in who's really over-weight. That's the elephant in the room, right? You all need to be comfortable running towards the danger and addressing this with your patients. But when you have become comfortable talking about the NEED to exercise, what are you going to do about it? You aren't going to be the doctor who just says, "Mrs. Jones, you need to exercise more."

Done, that's it. On to the next, right?

No, that doesn't work.

Most of the public is lost in what they should be doing, and the vast majority of the American population thinks that exercising and working out consists of sitting on a machine and counting reps.

When someone is super overweight, you have to talk about it. One of the first things we ask our patients is, "What are you doing right now for exercise?" The concept of regular exercise needs to be such a normal thing in your clinical culture that the idea of not exercising should be a rarity, not commonplace. Until your patients develop a routine exercise schedule, you're really not going to be able to help them reach and maintain true health.

If someone comes to you and they're very overweight or even obese, I guarantee you, at some point, their M.D. or family practice doctor, has said to them, "You should think about losing weight or exercising." The doctor probably gave them no specifics whatsoever and didn't tell them anything helpful, and as a result, things usually didn't change.

So many times, we would see patients come into our clinic and they would say, "Yeah, I went to my doctor and they told me I have high blood pressure or something. And they told me that I need to exercise more." And that's great, but that's such a blanket statement to tell someone. This advice does very little to solve their problem, when these patients have pain and it hurts when they exercise. As a result, they don't really know where to begin.

It's like taking someone who has no background in mechanics and their car breaks down. They take their vehicle into their mechanic. The mechanic runs the diagnostics, and then they offer this advice as a solution:

"Well, you blew up the motor in your car. What you need to do is take your car home, and you've got to fix that motor."

THE END.

Can you give me some guidance? What's step one? What's step two? What kind of tools do I need to do it right?

This is what the general public really knows about healthy, functional exercise: very little.

Maybe someday, we can work towards a model in healthcare that addresses a movement-illiterate person with the same level of urgency and specificity, as they would for a case of appendicitis. A model in which doctors would see one's inability to move as a huge red flag, a precursor for future disease, disability, and premature death. This type of theoretical healthcare, if it ever happens in a mainstream model, would be one of the biggest solutions to turning our health crisis around in this country.

Earlier, we started talking about how, back in the day, people used to exercise much differently, and the facilities they used were structured more like a gymnastics center versus the majority of the gyms that you see today. And then, we all know Arnold Schwarzenegger. He was the face of the modern bodybuilding era. He started really getting bodybuilding well known across the board. How many machine-riddled gyms do you think are out there just because of the impact that Arnold Schwarzenegger made? How many people do you think originally became interested in weightlifting just because they saw Arnold and said, "I want to learn how to be like that"? One of the most famous bodybuilding documentaries ever made was called, "Pumping Iron." This film starred none other than the man himself, Arnold Schwarzenegger. The bodybuilding era was an absolute kick-starter to the future of fitness, but as in most models out there, it was one of the first attempts. And being the first, much improvement needed to be made.

So gyms started popping up all over the place. Initially, there were still many free-weight options in most gyms. Just like in

"Pumping Iron," there was a good number of squats and deadlifts, but it was definitely weighted heavier towards the muscle isolation, machine-assisted exercises. I think what started to happen is that people got excited about bodybuilding, and gyms started opening up. The public flocked to these gyms and people started getting hurt because they didn't really know what they were doing. They didn't go about things in the correct order. Instead, they just jumped right in. Maybe they didn't have the athletic background that Arnold and other people had, so the compound movement exercises like squats and deadlifts were used less and less, and that's when the machines started to take over. That's when we started to see the gyms pack more equipment into smaller spaces. You know, machines are hard to do wrong. Meaning, almost anybody can sit down and get going on the "pushy thing" or the "curly thing." If the equipment only allows the user to move the pierce in one direction, it's hard to mess it up. That's why we started to see gyms transform.

The worst part about the move towards the machines is that people usually didn't get hurt right away, as they could work out for several months, even years, and they would see the esthetic results and the strength gains. These fitness goals are based on an illusion that is supported by society. Biceps and six-pack abs equals health, even if they can't bend over and touch their toes. The esthetic aspect is like a badge of honor. "Oh, I'm so huge and so stiff I can't even turn around." I personally know this concept very well, because I lived it! Back in 2009, I caught the bodybuilding bug, and my goal was to get bigger and stronger, with no real end in sight. I was about 35 pounds heavier than I am now with 6 percent body fat. I did lots of heavy lifting, and I ended up tearing a tendon in my elbow. I was very dysfunctional. I had to literally warm up my triceps for 15 minutes before I ever did any bench-press or overhead press because I had such bad triceps tendonitis. I had trained into all this dysfunction, and I was reinforcing movement patterns that led to an injury. With this style of training, some people get injured right away. And that's a blessing, as the problem is identified early on in this quest for fitness, with ample time to change course and prevent any major injuries.

In many cases, it can take five or six years of this repetitive style of training before an injury emerges. This type of exercise breeds stiffness, immobility, and dysfunctional movement and screws up the motor control aspect of things, such as how the brain coordinates and regulates movement patterns. If you don't identify these problems and learn how to reverse the damage that has been done, you're setting yourself up for a lifetime of problems, future surgeries, chronic pain, and disability. In the bodybuilding scene, the idea of dysfunction was not even a factor. It wasn't on the radar at all.

Conversely, you had a part of the population that didn't like weightlifting, and they turned to things like yoga. When I asked Tony to chime in on this topic, he had this to add:

"I was very lucky when I started as a personal trainer. It was in the early 2000s, when yoga really started to take off, and I was in New York City at the time and everyone was into it. We had yoga classes at my gym and there were yoga studios. And I would talk to people about why they were doing it. One of the things they always said is that they liked the way that it made them feel. There was this idea that if you could get more flexible, you would be healthier and stronger. Yoga was the perceived answer. Not to mention, a lot of people out there didn't like doing cardio or lifting weights, so this was an alternative thing that was attractive to them. I think the reason people experienced such improvement was because, if they applied the practice of yoga correctly, it's in some ways very similar to a functional movement model in which the practitioner is moving in multiple planes of motion and experiencing different positions that are very helpful for strengthening but also maintaining their flexibility."

Now, as a chiropractor, there are certain things I appreciate with many forms of yoga and some I do not. Yoga, like anything else, is not a cure-all for everything. Without knowing the alignment or quality of one's spine, simply throwing flexibility at it can sometimes result in disaster. Some of the worst spines I've ever seen in practice are the people who stack excessive mobility (flexibility) on top of an abnormal structure. I remember this patient a few years back. She was a yoga instructor, an older lady probably in her late 60s. She came in complaining with sciatica and I remember she said something to the extent of, "I don't know why I have this pain. I do yoga every day. I have such great flexibility." We took X-rays and I had some significant findings. For one, a complete lumbar kyphosis! So her lumbar spine was going the wrong way. Her spine was riddled with severe osteoarthritis. Her body was breaking down dramatically. I explained to her that she has developed all of this mobility and flexibility but she didn't have a stable structure to begin with.

Tony added this perspective: "Out in New York, within a couple years of yoga getting popular all of a sudden at my gym, we saw that most injuries were not people doing squats and biceps curls but taking yoga classes. There's a lot of people who would say, 'Oh no, I hurt my hip. I hurt my back. I hurt my neck.' They're doing stuff that's way out of their capability, like trying to do headstands or stuff like that. And they're not ready for it. Or like Dr. Todd said, they had some sort of dysfunction that was hidden but flared up when they started doing yoga."

That's where looking at spinal curves on an X-ray and understanding alignment becomes so crucial in really understanding the whole picture, including one's movement. I feel very strongly that we, as chiropractors, must own the understanding of functional movement. After all, in my opinion, we should have all of the necessary tools (this goes for the exceptional chiros, not the slackers). Skilled chiropractors have a thorough understanding of biomechanical assessment, X-ray analysis, and the ability to dive deeper in looking at the segment, posture, and movement. This is something that we will absolutely touch on in this book.

So, as we wrap up yoga, our next topic on the list is Cross-Fit. These two models have many pros that are not found with the machine model of fitness. CrossFit, especially, was one of the first mainstream fitness practices that started to popularize the shift where we are now, focusing more about full-body functional movement.

"The first rule of CrossFit is you have to talk about CrossFit." There are so many memes and jokes and things online about Cross-Fit, but few can deny they have created more than just a way to exercise. They have created a worldwide culture. You have people around the world who have opened up these gyms (called "boxes"), and in order to use the CrossFit brand and curriculum, they pay a franchising fee back to headquarters. These group-training-style fitness centers attract people like by the busload. They want to get in and start moving, no matter what.

Some of these "boxes" are better than others. There are the facilities in which the trainers or the gym owners really understand a great screening process, so they're not haphazardly exposing some of their beginner clients to exercises or movements that are not appropriate for their level of movement capacity. Conversely, there are the "boxes" that take the approach of, "Oh you've never worked out a day in your life. Come on in. Let's do some overhead deep squats on day one." And guess what happens. They get injured. We see many patients that share this story of injury. This inspired us to create this entire branch of our MoveWell University program, where we go out in the community and connect with the local gyms and fitness facilities, called "Marketing MoveWell." We will touch on that later down the road, in this book.

I think this is a good start to discussing the evolution of exercise, which, in just a few decades, has gone from a muscle isolation model to more of a full-body, Olympic lift for some type of group training. Each one of these approaches has its fair share of concerns and potential injury-producing consequences. In my opinion, these different methods all have one thing in common for the chiropractic clinician. They reinforce the importance in our craft — understand-ing spinal curves, spinal structure, and the quality of joints before one jumps into loading all of these movement patterns. The need for a more in-depth screening process becomes more apparent. With that said, the trends in exercise and fitness that move further away from the muscle isolation model are definitely on the right track. So hats off to them on that.

The next thing we're going to talk about is the current state of exercise.

CHAPTER 2

What Is Functional Movement?

The Current State of Exercise

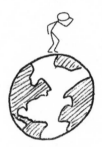

I N THE PREVIOUS CHAPTER, WE COVERED THE EVOLUTION of exercise. It's a little bit of a longer chapter, but we discussed some foundational basics to hopefully get you more interested in this exercise conversation, to see the need for the chiropractor to be involved in this arena. In this chapter, we will cover the current state of exercise. What in the world is going on right now in the world of exercise?

This is cool because I feel that we have a different perspective on the topic. I'm a chiropractor. I'm just like so many of you readers going through this book. My cohort on this, Tony, has been a personal trainer for over 15 years, so he's seen a lot of stuff. Ultimately, we're in the trenches working with patients each week, implementing these clinical approaches, and reporting back to you what is working and what we have changed to work even better.

When I asked Tony his take on this, he had this to say:

"As Personal Trainers, we love certifications. On one hand, we need to get them anyway for continuing education, and on the other hand, we love having a nice big toolbox of all this cool stuff that we can turn to in order to get better results with our clients. It was really interesting to me to see how the classes and certifications that were popular in the personal training world really covered a wide variety of topics. Earlier in my career as a personal trainer, it seemed to be more popular to see seminars and certifications that covered Olympic lifting. Then it became popular to see things being offered to personal trainers that covered more clinical therapy-type things: learning about trigger point therapy and proprioceptive neuromuscular facilitation (PNF) stretching. It started to be a lot of stuff that we used to think was only in the area of physical therapy, but we were learning something basic that we could handle and when it was appropriate to refer out to a physical therapist. If somebody had some sort of serious problem with their shoulder or their hip or something like that, we had a protocol for sending them out to the PT. Now, it was in their hands.

For me, it was about developing my toolbox. Throughout my years in the personal training world, I have definitely seen my own evolution. When I started out, I came into this similar to how Dr. Todd did. One day I was focused on the bodybuilding model. There was arm day, chest day, and all that kind of stuff. As I developed experience working with a wider variety of clients, things began to change. It became obvious that I needed to expand my horizons, and that's when I started getting into kettlebells, bodyweight exercises, yoga, martial arts, and all of that kind of stuff.

I felt that I had a greater ability to progress or regress stuff as much as I needed to. For many, taking exercise back to the fundamental basics. I had many clients who were a little bit older and had not been actively doing a whole lot of movement. I was able to apply my knowledge and quickly come up with stuff for them to do that was appropriate and useful.

Fast forward to what we're seeing now, clinically. If you understand the big picture, you can take someone, whether they're a beginner or an advanced athlete, and put together a methodical approach to movement progression that doesn't just aim to correct the dysfunctions that may be causing pain or a resulting injury, but also progress them to a point to improve fitness and athleticism, really addressing their overall health."

Ok, so we have jumped right to the functional movement discussion, but I realize that we still haven't even really defined the term "functional movement," so this is a good time to talk about it briefly. We just did a training last week for our exercise staff. One of the questions that I was asking one of our newest exercise therapists after she'd been training for a couple of weeks was, "How would you explain to a patient what functional movement is?"

To my delight, she did a pretty decent job answering the question. She went on to say:

"Here's how I would explain it. I would actually ask them a question first. I would say, 'Have you ever been a baby before? Was there ever a time in your life that you were a baby?' That's how I would start the conversation to make people laugh, to make it funny. From there I would ask, 'Ok, well how did you learn how to walk and how did you learn how to roll over? Or how to crawl?' I would try to get them thinking a little bit and then go from there."

Throughout the training, I helped further the conversation. I explained that they could then talk about the sequential order of movements that we all learn when we're an infant, growing into a toddler. First, we start off in the lying position, and if we're lucky our parents put us face down because the research has shown that infants who are placed in a safe, facedown position during these early developmental phases possess a higher IQ. Next, as we develop, we begin to start to roll over, and then we progress into a quadruped (hands and knees) position. We progress to crawling and then we get a little braver. We may progress to some tall kneeling positions or even jump straight up into walking. Then we try out running and jumping, and we are off to the races.

So, in addition to the above example of how our staff communicates these concepts to patients, this is also a great platform to explain why functional movement matters to begin with and how this all feeds back into human development. Another point to bring up to patients is calling attention to how children naturally bend and move throughout their environment. They will not default to the dysfunctional and dangerous movement patterns that we see with so many adults, such as bending at the low back and flexing at the spine in a dangerous pattern. Instead, children will typically get up close to an object and either deadlift or squat down in order to pick it up in a fairly functional capacity. These patterns of movement that we possess as children should remain intact for the rest of our adult lives.

As the science and awareness of functional movement developed over the last few years, there have been a handful of offshoots that present their take on the topic. One of the variations focuses on "primal movement." Their system consists of rolling, crawling, and climbing, movements that do not require any resistance other than one's own body weight. The concept of needing to practice these primal movement patterns stem from a deficiency created by a society that revolves around sitting and stagnation.

As if we haven't given you enough good reason yet, let's cover why one should engage in functional movements? Simple. That's what will prevent injury. Practicing functional movement will keep one more flexible and mobile, as well as keep their body healthier, their spine healthier, and their joints healthier, and it will increase the odds of living a long, healthy life. Some of the healthiest people alive are those who have lived a life that revolves around being able to move. Some of the most well-known health gurus, like the Juiceman, Jay Kordich, have made flexibility and exercise a priority in their daily life. Early on in a patient's care, sometimes, I will work this concept into their health goals, by asking them a question. I will say something to the effect of, "How much longer would you like to live?" They oftentimes reply with something like, "Well, if I'm hurting like this, I don't want to live that much longer."

I would then probe further saying, "What if you weren't hurting and if you were mobile and you could live a long, healthy life to meet your great, great, grandkids? I mean that's would be rewarding, right?"

So people settle on these limitations, assuming that this is an accepted norm, because they can't move well, their posture is failing them, and their joints are painful and arthritic. Ultimately, all of these variables come back to the importance of achieving and maintaining functional movement. Engaging in functional movement is the answer to living a long, healthy, and mobile life that is free of joint pain and arthritis.

To summarize this chapter, I defined functional movement and I focused on discussing the quality of movement. Remember, it's quality not quantity. It's better to do a qualitative and healthy movement than go through a sub-par movement over and over again. And then, in the last part, I mentioned getting people moving well and then having them move well more often. In the next chapter, I will talk about is the limits to the current models including chiropractic care and physical therapy.

CHAPTER 3

Limits to the Current Model

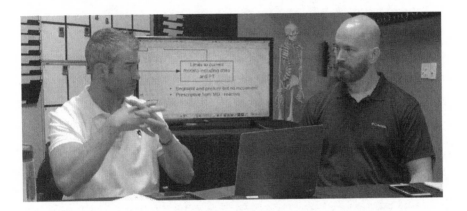

I N THIS CHAPTER, WE'RE GOING TO TALK ABOUT THE LIMITS to the current models of healthcare, including chiropractic care and physical therapy.

Tony shared this story: "Before I started as a personal trainer, I had really bad posture, and I was very kyphotic. I remember going to my family doctor because I started lifting weights and my shoulder started hurting. And he told me that I needed to stop lifting weights, which is not what you want to hear as a personal trainer. I was lucky enough that he referred me to a physical therapist, who explained that my problem wasn't the weightlifting. It was my posture. She said that if I fixed my posture, I could go back to weightlifting. I paid attention."

Tony continues: "Fast forward to a few years later, when I became a personal trainer. Unfortunately, not a lot had changed, but I was lucky enough to develop a relationship with one chiropractor and one physical therapist, in particular. I was confident that these two practitioners were not going to use that same line with my clients, unless something really major was going on. And I knew they would consult with me and keep me in the loop. As a personal trainer, when you're taking your client through their workout and they report feeling pain on a regular basis, this is a red flag that triggers a referral. That's exactly why it's nice to have a network of doctors, chiropractors, and physical therapists you can trust who are not going to take your business away."

Tony's views on these topics have been instrumental in the development of a program that I built called "Marketing MoveWell." This is a whole section in MoveWell University, which we discuss further in a later chapter. When we started building MoveWell University, we were designing this program to address trainers and fitness professionals. It didn't even cross our minds to share this with other chiropractors. At first, we put together a program we could teach to fitness professionals because we had really awesome stuff to share, and we knew we could help them. Initially, when I taught these seminars, I would go out to the gyms and the trainers were very enthusiastic about functional movement, but the problem was it took me so long to set up and teardown. It was taking me around two hours to set up and break down, in order to conduct a 90-minute workshop. I eventually changed the approach and invited trainers to our clinic, and there were times we would have five to ten trainers gathered together on a Friday afternoon to learn functional movement. This was an improvement from me going out to the gyms, as I saved the travel time and they were in my house (my clinic). Even with the trainers coming to us, the 90 minutes was barely scratching the surface of what they could take away and implement immediately. There was no way I was going to be able to go through and really give them the resources they needed in that amount of time. The goal was to teach them assessments, so they were better equipped to spot injury situations that would be appropriate to refer out. This is how we started working with fitness professionals, and this is what spawned the creation of what is now the MoveWell University for Fitness Professionals.

The idea that we came up with next was to help other chiropractors implement these systems of functional movement in their practices. Many chiropractors were addressing the segment, maybe even addressing posture, but they were rarely using systems to analyze or correct movement dysfunctions. We introduced the concept and the model that we use to explain how this comprehensive approach works together: segment, posture, and movement.

A lot of the things that we're sharing with you are not ideas or concepts that we just tried once and miraculously got right. Rather, these are systems that resulted from lots of trial and error. We failed several times before we finally found what actually worked.

When I first started in chiropractic, all I knew was the segmental approach. I believe this was an important place for me to start. This was my only intervention for a patient, so it had to be dialed in to the T. I focused on the Gonstead system, and the way that this was presented was this system had the ability to fix almost anything under the sun, solely by adjusting the subluxated segments in the spine or the extremities. I followed that mantra, and I carried this into practice for several years. On one hand, that was helpful, as it forced me to put 100 percent of my effort into the skill of assessing and adjusting the spine. On the other hand, this mindset kept me sheltered from any and all rehabilitation interventions out there. I had my blinders on, refusing to entertain anything beyond the adjustment.

Knowing what I know now, I see that there is a need for a rehabilitative approach in order to help stabilize and correct the underlying problems that we see with so many of our patients. By telling a chiropractic student that the adjustment alone will correct all of the underlying issues they will see in a patient is a gross oversimplification, and it is simply not accurate. I do feel that a specific chiropractic approach yields better results than a gross, global approach. However, the posture and the movement component cannot be ignored.

The funny thing I've found is that every technique system likes to believe that their system is the "magic bullet." When I was seeking out a postural and curve-correction approach, I turned to the Chiropractic BioPhysics Seminars. This system has published the most research. Their style is very detailed and methodical, and this method resonated with my principles. Just like so many other techniques, they present the postural approach as the "most important component."

I remember when I went to my first CBP seminar in Park City, Utah. The topic was "Thoracic Rehabilitation." I felt like a kid with a shiny new toy, so I was in awe as the presenters shared clinical cases and showcased the comparative X-rays where they were transforming the shape of their patients' spines. I saw these interventions as the ultimate solution for all of the things I felt I was still missing in practice. The CBP group presented their approach in the same way as so many other technique systems. My impression, after attending the first seminar (and dozens thereafter), was these interventions will fix everything under the sun. If the posture is fixed, the function is improved, because, as they repeated over and over, "structure dictates function."

The posture and curve-correction methodology teach that if the patient has a spine that is aligned and curved within a range compared to an "ideal" model, this person is considered to have a structurally sound spine. And further, it is implied that this will carry over into their functionality. This isn't always the case.

Let me first provide an example of how this IS the case. Let's say a middle-aged woman has a thoracic hyperkyphosis, or too much mid-back curve. Let's further say that it is a rigid hyperkyphosis. Her structure will NEVER allow her to go into a functional, healthy extension movement pattern. When she tries to extend backwards, she will move excessively in her thoraco-lumbar spine and likely move too much at her lumbo-sacral region. Her thoracic spine will not be contributing as it should. Her structure will hinder her function, and this will show up in her movement. In this woman's case, she could very well improve her extension pattern as her thoracic hyperkyphosis is addressed and reduced, like with traction and postural corrective exercise. We see this all of the time.

Now let's provide an example of the opposite scenario. You have a middle-aged man with a spine that is straight from the front, no shifts or deviations. Further, on the side view, his head, ribcage, and pelvis all line up and balance one atop the other. His sagittal curves are also within normal limits, approximately 40 degrees or so in his lumbar, thoracic, and cervical spine. This same man experiences a low-back "episode" a few times per year. When he bends forward to tie his shoes, he locks up in this position and can't move. He is injured.

He presents to your office. You analyze his posture and spinal integrity, and it all checks out. So how could this man have a problem? His spine is "ideal." Upon a movement assessment, you will find that when he flexes forward, he has a very tight posterior chain. He says that he feels tight in his calves, his hamstrings, and his low back. When he is asked to demonstrate some very basic core challenges, like a standard plank, he is unbelievably weak. So what has happened here? He lacks core stability, and his brain has taken over in an attempt to brace and protect his spine when he flexes forward. It does this by creating stiffness and tightness in his posterior chain — his calves, hamstrings, and lower back. This attempt to create stability only lasts for so long, and a few times a year, his body fails when he simply bends forward to tie his shoes. His lower back instability finally taps out, and he irritates a disc. But he has a great-looking posture, his alignment is within normal limits, and his sagittal curves are all there, so how can this be? This is an example of how structure alone is not enough. A sound structure does not ensure that one's functional movement is adequate.

I'm sharing these above examples, because it has become very apparent to me, in order to really help our patients to the fullest extent, we MUST be addressing both the structural component AND the functional component.

STRUCTURE VS. FUNCTION

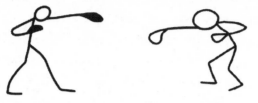

It's extremely important to address posture because the patient will hit roadblocks with their movement exercises. Movement interventions alone will not provide the total solution for their condition. If the patient has a cervical kyphosis or a lumbar hypolordosis or even worse a lumbar kyphosis, you need to address that posture with traction, postural corrective exercises, and spinal adjusting (and, at times, extremity too).

In the above case, it doesn't matter how much movement corrective intervention that you do, you're not going to fix them until you start to remodel the shape of the spine in the normal direction. You must understand this patient's limitations due to their abnormal structural issues, so that you can modify their movement expectations.

When I was primarily focused on the structural component alone, I was still practicing in New Mexico. One of my colleagues, who was also a devout Gonstead practitioner, got into exercise and functional movement around the same time that I got into the postural approach. I was in the "posture camp," while he was in the "movement camp." This created some tension, some arguments, and some competition.

We both thought we were right and the other was wrong. I remember when he would have a patient who just overcame a huge clinical milestone, and he would showcase the movement-based approach that he used. This other doctor would make a point to tell me that he didn't need to use any traction or postural corrective exercises, and he did indeed demonstrate some great improvement and structural changes.

And I, on the other side, would be quick to show him the newest set of comparative X-rays of my patient, where the patient had a cervical kyphosis. And on the follow-up X-ray, the cervical curve was now lordotic in a much healthier position. I would point out how I used traction and why that was so important.

Years later, looking back at how we both flexed our clinical opinion, I realized that we were both wrong. Neither one of us had the entire story.

Soon thereafter, my wife and I relocated to Idaho. This is where I furthered my knowledge and clinical experience using Chiropractic BioPhysics, but I still felt like something was missing. I would take care of patients who had alignment and curves that were pretty close to the "ideal" model. Being that I was laser-focused on posture, I would focus on the really subtle deviations, or curve discrepancies, with traction and postural corrective exercise. I would prescribe a traction setup for a spine that had a slight decrease in the neck curve, or maybe a very small deviation to the side of the head compared to the ribcage. I was so focused on the small details that I was missing something big. I wasn't addressing the main cause of their problems.

That's when I started studying the movement aspect, and that's when I realized how much I really didn't know. One can solely dedicate their entire life to studying functional movement. It's a topic that can go into great depth and specificity. I will cover this more in later chapters. Implementing functional movement can be a little intimidating and prevent people from diving in. Initially, that was a major deterrent for me as well.

I was eager to add a movement component to our clinical approach, and I asked myself, "Where do I begin?" I began looking for a program that was tailored to chiropractors to teach the protocols surrounding measuring and correcting movement and how to put it into practice. I needed to find a system that covered the various components involved in implementing this type of exercise department, the clinical side of things, how to communicate these concepts to the patient, and how to make it compliant. I also needed to know how to properly document so I could bill insurance and get reimbursed. A program like this just didn't exist, which is why I created MoveWell University.

I've spent several years, a lot of my own time outside of the clinic, tens of thousands of dollars, and many weekends travelling all over the country to acquire the resources necessary to build a top-notch exercise department in our clinic. For those out there who are interested in learning what it takes to do this right, MoveWell University will be a huge benefit.

Moving on. Let's switch gears and talk about how most healthcare practitioners look at these movement-related issues and how they are referring their patients out to other specialists. The relationship between medical doctors and physical therapists is interesting. As I have gone through various movement-related seminars, I have had the opportunity to meet and befriend a few very skilled physical therapists. I wanted to understand their perspective on how they feel in the healthcare model, and they all shared a similar sentiment, one of frustration.

The unanimous perspective of the handful of physical therapists that I surveyed was as follows: They feel "handcuffed" as far as how they treat their patients, as most of these PTs are not necessarily creating their own treatment plans for these people. What that means is a common practice in the MD-to-PT referral process is that the MD calls the shots. They send over the referral. They make the diagnosis. They dictate the duration of care. The PTs want to maintain the ongoing MD referral, as this, in most cases, is their primary vehicle for seeing new patients. So the PTs don't rock the referral boat, they feel as though they need to come across as grateful for what they are getting. Keep your head down, keep working, and don't question anything.

The therapist may absolutely want to progress their patient to a full-body movement pattern intervention, but they can't. The MD "gave" them 12 visits and outlined what they want the therapist to focus on the shoulder pain. The treatment is designated to the shoulder problem, so that's all the therapist can do. What if the patient has a thoracic spine issue that precedes the shoulder issue or an overbearing lower-extremity issue that would greatly benefit the patient's overall fluidity of movement and stability? This co-management between MDs and PTs has evolved into a very dysfunctional relationship.

In the above scenario, the patient ultimately suffers. I think that MDs are reluctant to refer their patients to a chiropractor for several reasons. They don't really understand the broad scope of practice that chiropractors possess. They don't realize that DCs are able to dig deeper into the diagnostic realm, especially those who have a more advanced understanding of spinal biomechanics and imaging. And lastly, I believe that many of the MDs like having control over the treatment plan, and they don't want to relinquish that control by referring to a chiropractor. With all of that said, I have also seen MANY medical doctors become open to supporting a MD-to-DC referral relationship, once they are exposed to a specific chiropractic approach that makes sense to them. This is what we have seen first-hand in our clinic.

Many movement practitioners may be of the opinion that functional movement should primarily be handled by physical therapists. The reality is even if the majority of PTs are trained in the background of functional movement, few are actually practicing in their clinical setting. They may not be setup to handle these types of movement-based protocols. Now, conversely, if you were a chiropractor who only wanted to focus on the adjusting portion of patient care, then you could always seek to develop a relationship with a physical therapist who is proficient in functional movement. That could be easier said than done.

So if you wanted to outsource the functional movement part to a physical therapist, that's better than pretending this component isn't important. In my opinion, a superior approach would be to keep all of this case management under one roof. This reminds me of the saying, "When you have more than one cook in the kitchen, the food starts to taste like garbage." In my opinion, a huge advantage to the chiropractor running the show is, as chiropractors, we have the ability to possess a more in-depth background and training in X-ray analysis and spinal biomechanics.

In addition, when something needs to be changed with patient care, it is helpful to be able to make these modifications on the fly instead of having the patient bounce around between multiple clinics.

So the moral of the story, for me, was that I wanted better outcomes. I strived for better results for my patients. You may be one who wishes to improve or add an exercise department in your clinic, or you may prefer to refer these patients to another provider. I think I make a compelling argument as to why you would want to handle this in-house, but either way, you should be familiar with this information. If your biggest hesitation to adding an exercise department has to do with space restrictions, there are solutions for this perceived hurdle as well. As a side note, when I first introduced spinal rehabilitation into my practice, when I was working as an associate doctor out in New Mexico, I cleared out a room we were using for storage and repurposed it to be able to render patient care. I have met several other doctors around the country who have taken a similar approach. Think about how you can be resourceful.

Again, my initial, ultimate driving force behind adding these other areas into my patient care was to improve my outcomes with patients. In my first several years as a chiropractor, I was addressing the segment-model only. Years later, I implemented the postural corrective approach, but I wasn't doing anything to measure or correct the movement aspect. Now, I am addressing all three in a structured, evidence-based fashion. The fact is if you have protocols in place for the segment, posture, and movement, then you are helping 90-plus percent of the patient population that will be walking through your doors. Sure, you will need to refer out periodically for special imaging or, in really rare scenarios, out to a surgeon for a surgical consult. But really, this has been a very fulfilling and exciting way to practice. As chiropractors, we have many advantages in the healthcare realm compared to other practitioners in this space. For example, the physical-therapy model is restricted, because, at least in most states, they don't have the authority to diagnose. They are basically given a diagnosis from a referring Medical Doctor.

From www.professionalpt.com: "In most states, physical therapists cannot make a medical diagnosis. ... While physical therapists are important members of your medical team, physicians are typically the healthcare providers that will provide you with a medical diagnosis."

Physical therapists also do not possess the training or permission to take or analyze an X-ray. In addition, as a standard, they do not learn about the spinal mechanics. They are not exposed to the in-depth postural analysis that exists in the chiropractic profession, and they do not have as detailed of a background in the basic sciences. I'm not saying this in any way to speak badly about physical therapists. I'm simply pointing out some of the differences in the training and the scope of practice for both of these professions. In the movement sciences, a large percentage of the advances that have been made can be attributed to the research and development conducted by physical therapists and strength and conditioning specialists.

Back when I attended a large movement assessment seminar, the audience was definitely PT dominant. There were maybe a couple of hundred people in attendance, and of those, three were chiropractors. I made friends with a couple of physical therapists at that particular seminar.

I remember I asked one, "So this is pretty common in physical therapy that all of the physical therapists have an advanced understanding of movement?"

He replied, "No, most of these PTs are only here so they can get their continuing education hours. The fact is that 99 percent of them will do none of this in practice. They're not set up like that and they don't have the time. They don't really care all that much and most of the care that they will do is dictated by medical doctors anyway."

As I mentioned before, I first learned about this functional movement stuff, and I was shocked that so few were doing this in practice. In my opinion, I feel that the chiropractic profession should be one of the leaders in bringing this to our communities. We should be working with fitness professionals, such as personal trainers, and branching out to pretty much anybody and everybody who deals with the community in the realm of movement. Think about it. That covers a ton!

This chapter helps summarize the limits of the current models within our healthcare system, as they pertain to understanding the movement component of human health. In the next chapter, we will introduce the curriculum that we designed, a program called MoveWell University.

CHAPTER 4

MoveWell University

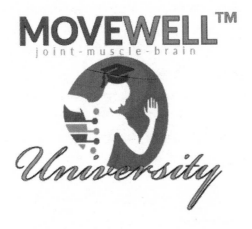

N THE LAST CHAPTER, WE TALKED ABOUT THE LIMITS TO the current models in the movement arena within the standard chiropractic approach and in the physical therapy profession.

We touched on the segment, posture, and movement components of care. In this chapter, we're going to talk about MoveWell University, which is the "pot of gold" at the end of the rainbow. You can get a ton of information out of this book, but I want you to think of the information we have been covering and will continue to cover as the "big picture," covering the background and diving deep into the principles behind the application. Conversely, MoveWell University is the application.

As you continue to read through this book, you will be left with a long list of action items that you will need to have at your disposal. You can either create these from the ground up, or you can use an organized combination that has already been tried and tested in clinical practice. This is MoveWell University.

The MoveWell University program was designed for those doctors who understand the importance of adding a corrective exercise department to their clinic but don't want to create every moving piece on their own. In order to save all of you chiropractors a ton of time and many of the challenges that go along with this type of endeavor, I created a turnkey system that just plugs into place.

Conversely, you may be the type of person who enjoys designing everything on your own, creating all of the paperwork, and trying and testing the systems until you get them right. If that's you, that's perfectly fine. This book will still provide you a framework to follow, so you do not miss the important components involved. With that said, we have found that most chiropractors appreciate the fact that we have done all of the heavy lifting for them, and they want to use their time more wisely. They choose to use MoveWell University to add or improve their current exercise platform.

MoveWell University is a very flexible system with what we call an "open architecture." It provides the framework and the steps involved to implement these systems, but it also has many areas that enable the chiropractor to customize this to their unique needs or practice style. In addition, it is important to note that this is our baby. Because of that, we will continue to nurture this program by adding more content and more value, and if we determine there is a better way of doing something within the current program, we will update that as well.

Within MoveWell University, we cover protocols, patient analysis, and patient engagement and put it all of this together in a smooth system. In addition, paperwork and documentation is a huge part of it. We touch on the compliance aspect as well as many of the communication concepts. The program has a built-in, automated marketing component that we will be talking about more in a later chapter, and we also make it easy to envision how this will fit into your current practice system and model. Even if you really don't know anything about functional movement or even exercise in general, MoveWell University makes it easy to learn and implement, because we have simplified and streamlined everything in order to save you time and money.

MoveWell University first teaches how to go through a movement screening that also doubles as an assessment. There is a difference between a screening and an assessment. The screening is a process to see if an individual is able to competently complete a minimum set of standards. The assessment is how you now determine why you are seeing any dysfunctions and figuring out which movement is less than functional. The MoveWell 3 accomplishes the goals of a screening, initially. The "advanced section" takes the practitioner through an assessment process.

Let me differentiate the concept of passive rehab versus active rehab. Passive rehabilitation is what you will find in most chiropractic clinics and many physical therapy offices. The patient has treatments applied. This serves a place in the clinical environment, but in the model aimed at addressing and restoring functional movement, the passive portion is only the beginning, not the end. The active component is the part that must be practiced in order to best serve the patient and correct their problem at its cause.

Another important concept that is addressed in the MoveWell University program deals with the human desire for transformation. The idea of transformation is really a big part of what we're doing here. We are getting our patients involved in this process of addressing and correcting their movement dysfunctions (as well as their posture and spinal health) and teaching them exercises and protocols they can do in the office and at home. In order for a patient to get the best results, they must follow our recommendations and be consistent. Our aim is to motivate our patients to find this inspiration within themselves, and we do this very effectively by focusing on setting goals. One of the most important steps that we cover on the "Day

Four" process — we have a four-day process with a new patient — is helping coach our patients to set health goals and then write them down. We help our patients set and write down both their 12-week, short-term goals, as well as their 12-month, long-term health goals. This is written down in the beginning section of a printed health journal that each of our patients receives. They are encouraged to bring this journal in with them to every single visit moving forward. This is part of our "12 Week Transformation" online membership site, which will be discussed more in a later chapter.

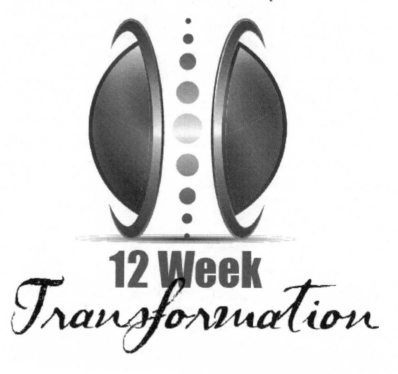

Some people have never written down health goals before (or any goals for that matter) in their entire life. This is why we coach them through the goal-setting process.

There is a saying regarding the doctor-patient relationship that is a bit surprising at first. It goes like this: "It matters less that your patients like you. What matters most is that they respect you."

When your patients respect you, they will choose you as a leader, and they will follow your guidance. Ultimately, that is in their best interest, as they will yield the best results.

I remember the first time I was exposed to the concept of goal-setting. I thought it was kind of cheesy to sit down and write goals. Honestly, that was something that existed inside my own headspace. I later learned that the act of physically writing down goals is one of the most powerful action steps that an individual can take to improve their likelihood to follow through with what they say they are going to do. These written goals are what the patient can reflect back on when they are tired or they've lost motivation, especially once their initial complaint or pain has gone away.

Tony adds, "I know, for me, as a personal trainer — and it's the same thing with chiropractic or other types of healthcare professionals — the first time you see the patient, they're going to start talking about why they've come to see you. So it's not weird to me to start setting goals in the very beginning. This is so effective. I think once you get used to setting goals, it doesn't seem as strange as it might at the beginning."

The goals we are helping our patients set are not to just fix the initial symptoms they came in for, but they are aimed at getting them to see their problem is a small piece of a much bigger picture.

Let's discuss the concept of prevention versus transformation. In general, most people really don't care about prevention. They need something more to motivate them to stick with a new habit or program. People are drawn to the idea of a transformation. People want to feel transformed, especially in a healthcare setting. They want to see and feel results, which is why functional movement is so powerful. Functional movement will help your patients experience and physically feel a transformation sooner, and it will allow them to further this transformation process in the comfort of their own home.

If you have been following what is trending on many reality TV shows, you will notice that people value transformation, and they want to be transformed quickly. One of my favorite shows is called "Flip or Flop," where a couple buys run-down houses and fix them up to sell for a profit. They come into a beat-up house that's growing mold on the walls and has flood damage, and they buy it for a low price. Through their trials and tribulations, they overcome. Finally, they make a huge profit and everyone is happy. People love that kind of stuff. That's what the public is attracted to. So why not speak to this concept of transformation in a healthcare model? You should.

We all see patients with the following story. They come in to see you on day one with low-back pain. As you go through their health history, you predictably discover that when they bend over to tie their shoe, this was simply "the straw that broke the camel's back." Or they tell you that they were pulling weeds in their backyard and it screwed up their lower back. The reality is they have been dysfunctional for a long time and something would eventually push the limits and test the waters. In order for your patient to see the value in their care, you have to be able to get them realize they were fragile and frail and this was inevitable. It was going to happen eventually. They need to say, "If I don't change my life right now, this is going to happen again and again. And it's going to get worse."

For many people, until they suffer one of these episodes themselves, they will never quite understand the need to make a change. People need to first experience what they don't want, so they can set a goal and take the actions necessary to get where they need to be. To be most successful in accomplishing this, they need to set goals.

Tony explains, "When I was a personal trainer, invariably, I had people come to me who were immediately ready to invest the time and the money to sign up for personal training. They knew that they would be investing the time and the money, but they had a strong desire to get out of the current situation they were in. These people, generally, had already gotten to a point where they knew they had to take some drastic action. For instance, they tried working out on their own or working on their diet by themselves, and they recognized that they needed help. And I think it's a similar situation in healthcare."

Now let's talk more about MoveWell University. We covered a little bit about how and why we put this together. We created this program to primarily discuss and teach chiropractors about functional movement. MoveWell University is a lot of the mechanics one could use to get this launched and operational in their practice. It's a step-by-step process, and it begins with covering the history of exercise and understanding why this history matters. Then we familiarize the chiropractor with the other movement screenings and assessments out there. We discuss the Functional Movement Screen (FMS) and the Selective Functional Movement Assessment (SFMA). This provides some background and context on where we're coming from and why we developed things the way we did. Then we pretty much hit the ground running from there. Like I said before, it's pretty straightforward. If you're a chiropractor who has joined MoveWell University and you are beginning to study the modules, the nice thing is that you really don't need to possess a background in this topic in order to jump right in and very easily get your feet wet.

There are several flowcharts in MoveWell University, which Tony created, since he is the "flowchart king." One of the challenges, when building a program like this, is determining how to take all of the stuff we learned that pertains to functional movement and intertwine it with chiropractic and present in an easily digestible fashion. One of our goals was also to make the assessment protocols powerful, effective, and time-efficient. It can be challenging for a chiropractor to perform a 30-minute assessment in the clinic with every single patient. We have developed a process that delivers a ton of information, and it can be performed in as little as five minutes for a simple case and under 15 minutes for a more severe, complicated case.

Tony adds, "We originally were going develop this MoveWell University for personal trainers, and we talked a lot about how I felt like the people who would most benefit were the trainers who were brand-new to the industry. And those were the same people who maybe didn't have the experience or the knowledge base to understand some of the more complicated stuff. From the beginning, we built this program in a way that's very easy to understand and implement. In the beginning, we had this content and format geared towards trainers, and then we realized this was so invaluable to other chiropractors, so we shifted our focus and continued to build this with the doctor in mind."

There's also a whole marketing aspect we created because as a MoveWell Doctor becomes an authority in their area, they can branch out and develop relationships with personal trainers and other fitness and movement professionals. The chiropractor can build this relationship by teaching periodic seminars to these movement professionals. One of the goals of this relationship is for the fitness professional to learn how to identify a stopping point with their client — whether it is pain, injury, or observed dysfunction. Then they can refer the client to the chiropractor when appropriate. Thanks to a coordinated team approach, the client can be properly clinically managed and able to safely returned to training.

In MoveWell University, we teach an assessment that we created called the MoveWell 3. When developing this assessment, we sat down and spent a good part of a weekend game-planning and going back and forth on what should be included. We took the best of everything that we knew and added a couple of other things we felt were missing in other systems.

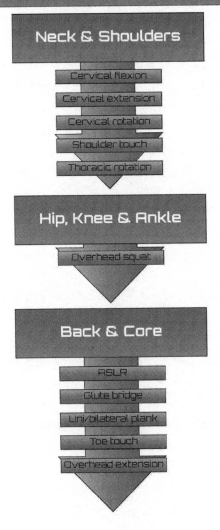

The MoveWell 3 Screening

Neck & Shoulders
- Cervical flexion
- Cervical extension
- Cervical rotation
- Shoulder touch
- Thoracic rotation

Hip, Knee & Ankle
- Overhead squat

Back & Core
- ASLR
- Glute bridge
- Uni/bilateral plank
- Toe touch
- Overhead extension

We came up with a six-minute process.

We then made videos of the entire process and went through it step by step. We made it super turnkey, where we break it down with flowcharts and explain how to fix certain problems if they arise. This style of flowchart systems is what I was looking for when I was designing my exercise department. It didn't exist, so I built it. My position on the need for this type of program was there are 10 million different exercises and progressions, but certainly, there's got to be some that work better than others. We identified the best protocols and then combined those into one system.

Tony explains, "Not only are a lot of the other assessments more complicated and more time-consuming, the interventions can send you down a rabbit hole searching for a simple solution for the patient. We've taken that thought process and really condensed it down and made it really straightforward. In fact, it's so straightforward that not only is this something a chiropractor with very little background in functional movement can implement, but they can turn this over to their staff, as long as they can follow step-by-step instructions."

The requirements vary by state, as far as the type of certification that your staff members need to assist in the exercise department and bill to a health insurance company. Some contracts refer to this position as a "service extender" or a "certified" individual. If you are billing a health insurance company, you must understand what the specific contract outlines and make sure you are abiding by their requirements. Oftentimes, the individual required to use for this position is one who may come in with very little knowledge in exercise, as they may be a Certified Medical Assistant (CMA). So how do you take someone like that and get them to understand this program? You make it simple yet comprehensive enough. And one of the cool things about MoveWell University is we have a system that gives an overview for how to train the staff. We share "The Belt System of Functional Movement," which beautifully organizes the progressive fashion of corrective exercise, once the chiropractor has prescribed the protocol prioritization. We have MoveWell Doctors around the country conduct a weekly staff training, using the MoveWell University training program as the teaching guide for these meetings.

In our clinic, we've had some new people join our team, and

getting them up to speed has become a much quicker process. We primarily use the membership site as their training portal for their first several weeks as a new employee. It's all very simplified and streamlined.

Before MoveWell University, I would spend many a weekend meeting with new exercise staff, training, and attempting to bring them up to speed as quickly as possible. I had recorded these trainings and assumed that these could be used for other staff, to leverage my time. That didn't work well, because how do you hand a three-hour video to a staff person say, "Here you go take notes and learn it"? This is how we started, and it was a frustrating endeavor. If we had hired somebody who ended up not being a great fit for the exercise position and we had trained them for a month, this was time wasted. We would have to let them go and started all over again from scratch with a new hire.

Utilizing the MoveWell University program as the primary staff training tool has saved us a lot of time. A second huge benefit is this also makes it less intimidating for a new hire to learn these systems, especially if they are new to exercise and fitness. Again, we recognize that the doctor's time is extremely important, so we share the same solutions that we used. The organized video library is vital for maximizing the staff training experience while demanding less time from the doctor.

Another major section that MoveWell University covers is all of the required paperwork that helps these systems flow smoothly. We have made nearly 20-plus revisions to every single piece of paperwork we have. We have a travel card and an exercise card that are used in the daily patient visit. In addition, we map out the patient's care with our recommendation card.

And then, on top of that, we go through the fee schedule system for insurance billing, as well as how our self-pay schedule works and how to use a compliant fee schedule through a company called ChiroHealthUSA.

As we discussed earlier, we use "The Belt System of Functional Movement" to organize the various exercise progressions. In addition, we designed an organized an exercise library inside MoveWell University. Due to popular request by so many of our original members, we even developed a set of "Pro" modules where we have video tutorials for our day one through Day Four systems, a communication module training to best handle objections, and an automated marketing module called: "Marketing MoveWell."

That's a brief overview of the MoveWell University program. If you are the type of person who prefers to build out all of these systems on your own, then this book will provide the most important variables to consider along the way. On the other hand, if you are the type of person who would rather use a tested and proven system for implementing or improving your exercise department, then MoveWell University is the solution for you.

CHAPTER 5

Societal Impact

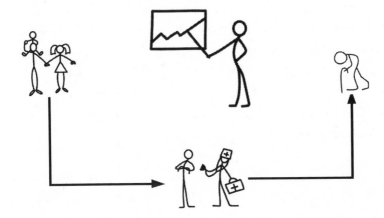

N THIS CHAPTER, WE'RE GOING TO TALK ABOUT THE SOCIE-
tal impacts of movement-related deficiencies. These impacts
pertain to the obesity epidemic, health outcomes, and overall
quality of life. In the last chapter, we talked about and the MoveWell
University program. I know that some of this seems repetitive, but I
try to present this from a variety of different angles so you are better
prepared for the conversations you will have in practice and throughout your community. When you begin to implement this in practice,
you have to know how to talk to people in a way that resonates with
their understanding, so they can see the value.

When you lead with the language of movement, this enables you
to reach and connect with many of those who may not be as open
to the topic of chiropractic. I'm not saying avoid talking about the

chiropractic message, but when I start with movement, in my experience, that is my foot in the door to places that otherwise would have shut me down.

Think of yourself as a pioneer. You are on the forefront of a healthcare revolution. When you begin to implement and master these concepts of functional movement, you will be responsible for changing the way that people think about their health and the healthcare model as a whole. The cost of healthcare continues to go up, and the costs of insurance premiums are astronomical. Tony and I often discuss how the healthcare model in the future is going to need to consist of people taking more personal responsibility for their wellness. We also believe that there will be a team involved in this process, consisting of healthcare providers, personal trainers, and other movement specialists who are going to teach people how to do that.

Sixty percent of the population is overweight, and we're getting close to 30-40 percent being classified as obese. In other words, the majority of our population is either overweight or obese. Does anybody else see this as absolutely crazy? Even though so many of these overweight individuals see their weight as a visual reminder on a daily basis, they commonly operate reactively instead of proactively.

For instance, think about flood insurance. People often wait to buy this type of insurance after there is a flood. Flood insurance is a prevention model. How does their health situation affect things they enjoy doing in their daily life? If the patient can't bend over and play with their children, but you can help them make an emotional connection with that movement deficiency and what that means for them now and in the future, then you can get through to them.

As a chiropractor reading this, realize that patients don't primarily come to see you because they have a pain or a physical problem. They come to see you because they can't do something they used to be able to do because of a physical problem. This is what you need to speak to as well:

"Mr. Jones, you said you can't play with your 3-year-old son because it hurts to bend down. That sounds frustrating."

The concept of incorporating a functional movement solution before a patient necessarily knows they have a problem is very powerful. Meaning, someone can be pain-free and think they are just fine. Then you take them through the seven different fundamental movement patterns. You demonstrate how they are not moving adequately, how there is a problem, and how this will cause even bigger problems in the future. You need to help them connect the dots. Once they understand why their low back "goes out" on them twice a year and their inability to demonstrate a functional and non-painful movement pattern actually means that they are a ticking time bomb, then they listen.

Once they begin to regain function, the next level is to help them set health goals that include strength, power, and fitness. This is what the healthcare model needs to be. If your patient isn't getting this somewhere, then they really aren't moving towards a true healthcare model. Why not make that "somewhere" your facility, under your guidance? In most cases, they aren't going to get this anywhere else, and if they do, pieces will be missing and the results will suffer. When this is all done in a congruent model, the outcomes are more meaningful and impactful.

Mind you, I didn't always practice like this. The majority of my time in practice, I was not addressing movement at all. I realize that my interventions in the past were not as powerful because of this missing component.

Without measuring and addressing movement with your patients, how long are your interventions going to last?

Not as long as they could. Especially when your patient leaves your office to go right back into prolonged sitting coupled with a sedentary home and work environment.

This is what hits home when you communicate this with your patients. With so many of the chiropractors that we have helped implement corrective exercise, I have seen the same thing time and time again. They feel as though they can finally position themselves as a true wellness clinic.

Tony adds, "I think that's what we're going to start seeing in the future. And it's what we've tried to do here, and I think Dr. Todd has done such a great job. Do you know how often we talk about this and get comments from patients, when they initially come into our clinic and they're looking around, because they've never seen a chiropractor clinic like this one before?

And furthermore, they have never seen anything in healthcare that is anything like this. I think most people don't think to turn to a chiropractor for a movement-related problem. There seems to be a disconnect in understanding how chiropractic and movement actually go together. We marry these concepts very well here. I think the public perception is 'if I want guidance on how to exercise and do all the stuff, I'll go talk to a personal trainer.' While that could be good sometimes, the majority of personal trainers don't really know a whole lot about functional movement or what their client should be doing, especially when there is an underlying injury."

Let's discuss how most gyms get started with a client. As a general rule, if the gyms do any assessment at all, it's probably something very basic. Maybe they're going to do an overhead deep squat or something like that, but there's a ton of other basics that should be measured prior to ever throwing someone into a squat pattern.

The squat is one of the most complex movements. It's a triple-flexion movement: hip flexion, knee flexion, and dorsiflexion. The squat requires stability, mobility, and, at least, a very minimal level of strength. It's probably not the best idea to make this the sole movement assessment tool, and then try to develop a training plan from there. It's pretty insane. It's better than doing nothing, but not far from it.

The majority of the trainers we come in contact with do not have a very well-versed background in understanding how to systematically measure and correct movement. The ones who do are few and far between, but even they still need a healthcare practitioner (like a chiropractor) to co-manage and intervene when they identify an injury or come to a stopping point.

In most cases, many of the trainers will approach an injury or a dysfunction as, "Well, you can't do that, so let's take it to a machine." The role of a competent personal trainer should not be just a professional "rep counter," but someone who programs the routine, customizes, and, most importantly, measures movement capacity and has the know how to identify when their client needs help from a healthcare professional.

In summary, the main point that we want to hit home is that when you add corrective exercise to your practice and add the functional rehab component, this has a very powerful impact on your patients and your community. Now they are hearing a message from a "doctor," an authority figure. That carries a certain weight that can result in the patient finally taking action. Sure, other doctors tell their patients, "Your blood pressure is up, so you need to exercise," with no real guidance or actionable steps to get them going. So what is the result? The patient rarely takes action. In this case, you are teaching your patient the importance of building strength, power, and incorporating fitness into their lifestyle. Further, you are making sure they're not jumping into things that are going to hurt them. You are even trying to pair them up with fitness professionals in the community who can take them further, once you have ensured that they can safely proceed.

This model differentiates and has differentiated our clinic so much, which is apparent just taking a tour of our clinic.

Once you become proficient in these systems, you now also have a solution for your overweight patients, so you're not just telling them to "lose weight start exercising" without a starting point.

These systems are things that I felt were crucial to address in practice if we were going to categorize our clinic has a "wellness" center. I knew deep down inside that we had to address these things, especially since we named our clinic Gonstead Spine & Wellness.

So really, what is wellness?

Wellness includes a few main topics. If your patient is overweight, you need to address that component. Weight loss includes how to eat properly, and it needs to incorporate how to move properly. That movement part must then evolve into an exercise component, which I feel so many clinics are lacking. Doctors may tell a patient to go work with a trainer and "start exercising," as if regaining movement and exercise is just a super easy thing everybody can just jump right into. Patients need the guidance and will commonly fail to take action unless they are clearly coached through the process step by step.

It's not like you can take an out-of-shape person with dysfunctional movements and give them a series of exercises so they will instantly become healthy again. The question must be asked, "Why can't somebody move well?" This leads right into the next chapter, where we talk about the concept "Segment, Posture, and Movement." This model lays out how we present our unique approach to the community and our patient and how movement and chiropractic go hand in hand. We begin by focusing on and talking about the importance of movement and how this is such an important variable in one's health. Then we explain the importance of posture and how that aspect must be measured and addressed in order to get the best results possible. Then, we tie this back to where things initially break down (in most cases) on a segmental level. That is how we connect movement back to chiropractic — the model of segment, posture, and movement.

This chapter pretty much concludes the first module of this book. In this next chapter, I will switch gears and dive deeper into the clinical model that brings this all together.

CHAPTER 6

Segment, Posture, and Movement Concepts

Segment

Posture

Movement

I N THIS CHAPTER, WE'RE GOING TO COVER THE CONCEPTS of this three-tiered approach that we use in practice: segment, posture, and movement. This model has defined who we are as a unique and different approach to chiropractic and has helped build many successful relationships with other healthcare providers and movement professionals in our community.

Let's start with posture.

You have some different groups out there who look at posture, and I will openly admit, I am biased. I've gone through all the training and earned my Advanced Certification in Chiropractic BioPhysics, and I haven't seen anything else that's as meticulous or evidence-based in regards to spine modeling and "corrective care." I learned a detailed understanding of how to assess a patient's posture in their static stance, and I learned how to understand how X-ray plays a part in this equation. How is that going to reflect on their segmental alignment and their movement capability? Static posture can predict how a patient is going to move, to an extent. For example, if a patient's pelvis is rotated counterclockwise in comparison to their feet, when they squat, they "corkscrew" down and come back up, which is an injury waiting to happen. There's a reason for that, which could be a leg length inequality or an imbalance between gluteus-medius and Q L (which is like a sling on the opposite side). It could be a problem on the sagittal plane, but often, the sacroiliac joint is normally blamed. How many of you have adjusted the S.I. joint and seen these rotational pelvic postures go away in 100 percent of your patients? Eighty percent? How about 50 percent? Ok, ok, 20 percent? My conclusion after 15 years in practice: If you want to best help your patient, you must address posture with a specific postural corrective approach.

As chiropractors, you're already dealing with the segments. Some of you are addressing the posture as well, or maybe you're not (you need to be). But very few are utilizing a customized approach to movement. Most chiropractors I know practice with a global or segmental technique. Many are well-equipped to do things with the spine, extremities, or muscle to get their patient out of an acute phase as quickly as possible. If a clinic is offering rehab, most of them do passive modalities such as electrical stimulation, ultrasound, ice, and heat. Spinal decompression is a common thing, because you can put someone on a machine (which is really expensive and looks very fancy) and patients are charged a large premium. There is definitely a science behind spinal decompression. It's axial distraction with a pumping motion that can be helpful in certain disc issues, but it can also be a detrimental therapy in certain cases (an important thing that I discovered as I was exposed to the research and teachings in Chiropractic BioPhysics).

In the fitness industry, posture is RARELY part of any kind of assessment process, from a personal trainer's perspective. With so much focus on movement, personal trainers really aren't well-trained to assess posture and definitely do not have any scope of practice to address the segmental component. I did an interview with a very knowledgeable personal trainer friend of mine named Marshall. We published this interview on the MoveWell Podcast, and he talked about how he's gone through many certifications and all have something in common when it comes to referring a client out for an injury.

"If you spot an injury or if it appears someone is injured, refer them to a doctor."

According to Marshall, that's the universal message taught at a variety of these certification seminars.

How much do you want to bet the patient will be encouraged to stop training with that trainer? Instructed to halt their fitness and exercise? At that point, the patient doesn't know what to do. This has created a fear from the personal trainer's standpoint. They don't want to risk losing their client or being badmouthed by a doctor, so they are less willing to refer out. This is not a good system, and fortunately, we have a better way. Keep on reading.

Many physical therapists, even if they are passionate about movement and want to go through various assessments and corrective fixes with their clients, do work that's not dictated by ta referring medical provider, so they can't. If that referral comes from a practice that makes up 95 percent of their business, you can see how the physical therapist is going to do when he is told a patient can pay out of pocket to keep going (if that is even presented as an option, and from my experience, it seldom is). The thing I have yet to find (and this is nothing against physical therapy) is a practice that has a system like the 12-Week Transformation to help patients stay engaged and see the true value in the program. My position has always been as follows: Even if the insurance is exhausted or a medical referral was for eight visits, you have an obligation to the patient to educate them and motivate them to stick with it. Creating excitement and value for the patient is a critical step in keeping them going.

Very few physical therapists, although some of them may be trained in functional movement assessments, are doing this in practice. The majority are focusing on muscle-isolation exercises, post-surgical care, and honing in on a specific symptom that the patient presented with or was sent in for treatment by the referring medical provider.

From a chiropractic standpoint, Chiropractic BioPhysics is teaching the most detailed postural approaches. If you're just seeking a basic foundation to begin with, we briefly talk about posture in our program. Understanding it in more detail should be on your radar, though. You can't fully fix movement issues and stabilize the segments of the spine when someone's stuck in a posture where their head is sticks out three inches in front of their body. Posture needs to be a consideration.

I'm somewhat familiar with what they're teaching in chiropractic school now. I also work with a lot of students and recent graduates, so I get feedback from them. For the most part, the consensus is they're exposed to a little bit more of the corrective exercise and functional movement as compared to when I was in school, but it's still done on a very basic introductory level, and it doesn't put the pieces together. With MoveWell University, you can help just about anyone on the fitness spectrum. I don't care how athletic or how nonfunctional or dysfunctional a patient may be. As chiropractors, we can help them best progress to a superior state of health and wellness when we address the segment, posture, and movement.

CHAPTER 7

Experts in Movement

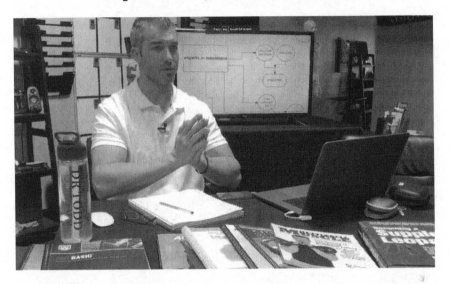

UNDERSTANDING THE DIFFERENT CONCEPTS OF SEG-
ment, posture, and movement are vital to incorporating
functional movement into a chiropractic model. The KEY
to effective functional movement protocols comes from the experts.

It's important to know the experts and understand what else is
out there in this arena. Some of the top players in the functional
movement arena are Lee Draper, Brett Jones, and Gray Cook. Gray
Cook and Lee Draper are physical therapists who are considered
the founders of the Functional Movement Systems (FMS). They
developed a widely used movement screening called the "Functional
Movement Screen." In addition, they developed a movement assessment to break down and diagnose the clinical variables, called the
"Selective Functional Movement Assessment" (or SFMA for short).

Let's briefly cover the difference between a screening and an assessment, to ensure we are all on the same page.

An example of a screening would an initial visual test using an eye chart. This is an example Gray Cook gives — he's the king of analogies. The eye chart is used to test how low on the line one can read, and that's it. This screening doesn't tell the examiner *why* the tester can't read a lower line. It simply identifies that there is a measurable deficiency. If the person being screened can only get to the third line down (which would not be very good), he would then go to a doctor who specializes in discovering *why* the measurable deficiency is present. The process of now measuring and diagnosing the reason for the less-than-optimal performance is the *assessment*. Does that make sense? Similarly, the FMS is the screening to see *if* a problem exists, the SFMA is for the healthcare professional to dig deeper and figure out *why* the problem exists.

Moving on with the experts, let me briefly introduce Brett Jones.

Mr. Jones is a Certified Athletic Trainer and Strength and Conditioning Specialist in Pittsburgh, PA. He is a master in Russian kettlebell work (he also happens to be the Chief Instructor of StrongFirst, a kettlebell group led by Pavel). Do a search on YouTube and you'll see all kinds of impressive "feats of strength" highlight reels. He demonstrates some truly impressive lifts with kettlebells, all the while emphasizing strength and power through a functional platform. Jones demonstrates how to develop and harness the power of the human body without causing injury.

Another name that should sound familiar to every chiropractor is Dr. Craig Liebenson, who is a chiro. He's well-known in the movement arena, and his name is often grouped with Gray Cook and Brett Jones. They don't necessarily work together on the same projects but they collaborate often. They each have their unique contribution to the science of functional movement.

Dr. Liebenson teaches seminars and has some great instructional videos out there. And he is a clinician, so he's practicing and seeing patients and sharing his clinical insight.

The next name that you need to know is Dr. Stuart McGill, Ph.D. Dr. McGill conducts research in the Spine Biomechanics Laboratory at the University of Waterloo. He has made several contributions to the movement sciences and has published many research papers in peer-reviewed journals. He is an intriguing lecturer and is well-known for defining various movement patterns that are limited or driven ones specific to anatomy. His concepts are really important to understand. He is a great guy to listen to. I recommend looking him up on YouTube. Dr. McGill has published several books. His most recent is "The Back Mechanic." It discusses differentiating functional tests to figure out what type of spinal injury you're dealing with, as well as the thought process behind how to best approach these different scenarios.

Another guy to check out is Brent Brookbush, founder of the Brookbush Institute of Human Movement Science. He is a physical therapist and has developed a substantial following with his instructional videos online. Brent is a natural teacher and has some great videos explaining different protocols and different soft-tissue techniques and assessment techniques to use in practice. I would recommend following his work as well.

Moving on to highlight popular names in the movement industry, you have a physical therapist and CrossFit gym owner Kelly Starrett. He wrote a book called "Becoming a Supple Leopard." Starrett is known as the "smasher." He has some interesting and effective self-manual therapy techniques that he outlines in his book. We have implemented several with patients in our clinical practice.

That's pretty much a summary of what I wanted to cover in this chapter, short and sweet. We touched on the various experts you need to be familiar with. In the next chapter, we will discuss the concept of functional fitness and some of the leaders in this area of the functional movement world.

CHAPTER 8

Functional Fitness

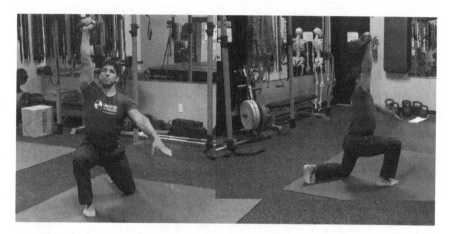

I N THE LAST CHAPTER, WE TALKED ABOUT EXPERTS WITHIN the movement arena. In this chapter, we're going to talk about Functional Fitness. Let's talk about this concept.

Functional Fitness is different than dysfunctional fitness. Functional Fitness means that you're doing something that reinforces healthy patterns. For example, there's a difference between a corrective exercise and a functional exercise. We go into in a lot of detail in our education portal and inside of the "Implementation" section of MoveWell University, our doctor training program. I'll summarize it here.

Let's say your problem is you can't move your shoulder properly. You're going to carry out interventions to regain normal shoulder range of motion and shoulder stability. You may include some isolated, corrective exercises that don't just aim to increase range of motion but focus on rebuilding a movement pattern. That pattern encompasses the coordinated movement between your scapula and your gleno-humeral joint. Those are corrective exercises (or activation exercises), scapular stabilization exercises, or shoulder packing, for example. To build on those gains, you'll want to evolve to strength, power, and fitness — what we call Functional Fitness.

Functional Fitness (functional exercises) reinforces healthy patterns. That's what leads to long-term improvement and maintenance. There are different styles of Functional Fitness exercises. Let's examine a few.

The first style is one that I've studied, I'm very interested in, and is how I workout myself. It is the work of Pavel Tsatsouline. Pavel brought Russian kettlebells to the US over 20 years ago. He was one of the first to popularize Russian kettlebells. Pavel's techniques have a large following. He is the leader of a group called StrongFirst. This group focuses on teaching strength and power techniques, primarily using kettlebells. They do some Olympic lifting-type of exercises and body weight strengthening work as well.

Brett Jones, who I talked about earlier, is StrongFirst's Chief Instructor, so you can rest assured that a master in the field of movement, strength, and power is overseeing this group.

Why should we care about kettlebells? There are all kinds of cool reasons why kettlebell exercises are such a great functional exercise technique for reinforcing health. In our clinic, we chose to focus on a set of Russian kettlebell exercises that we call the Functional Four. We use the Functional Four in patient care. We share them with other doctors, and we strongly suggest you make these a goal for your patients. In order to build strength and power, your patients should be to do at least some level of the Functional Four.

The Functional Four exercises are a progressive set. The first thing you're going to want someone to perform competently is the kettlebell deadlift. The second one is going a kettlebell swing. Next is the goblet squat, which is like a front squat. The fourth one is the get up. These are the Functional Four exercises. If your patients can do those completely, from start to finish, with a moderate amount of weight, these exercises will reinforce almost every functional movement pattern in the body.

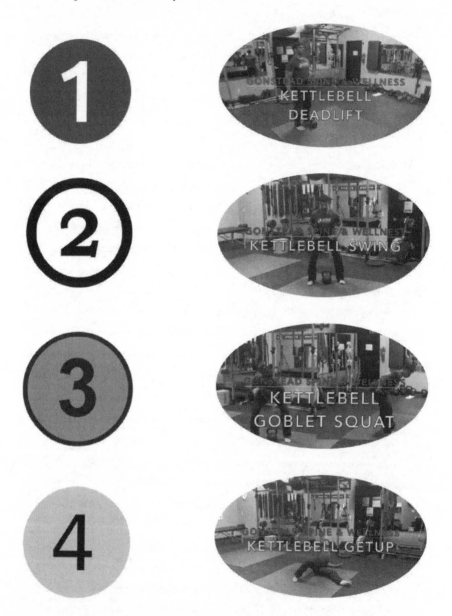

The "Functional Four," demonstrated by my great friend and kettlebell expert – Zar Horton, StrongFirst Master Instructor.

The beautiful thing about this is that if your patient can't perform these exercises, you can identify this pretty quickly. Now these benchmark four exercises can be used as part of the screening process, cuing the exercise therapist or clinician to backtrack and address some of these movement deficiencies before proceeding. The amount of weight used depends on the size and strength of the patient. The components that are required to properly execute these exercises include hip mobility, core stability, glute activation, shoulder mobility, scapular stability, coordinated cervical patterning, and posterior chain activation. There is a lot great stuff in the Functional Four. We can thank Pavel for bringing the Russian kettlebell to the United States.

A popular style of exercise that incorporates full-body movements is called CrossFit. You may have heard of it before (if not, it's likely you have been living under a rock). Whether you love it or you hate it (or are somewhere in between), CrossFit incorporates Olympic-style lifting techniques. There are a lot of routines they promote that include exercises such as running, jumping, and dynamic movements like box jumps and burpees.

I have some concerns about CrossFit. I don't think it's a good idea to do CrossFit exercises in high reps. And I don't recommend doing CrossFit exercises with the goal of trying to beat the clock at the expense of sacrificing proper body mechanics and form. As exhaustion kicks in, the form starts to get sloppy and that's where injuries occur. How CrossFit exercises are used depends on the style of the CrossFit trainer and of each individual. I think that CrossFit itself is on the right track, as far as looking at more compound functional movements for strength and power and fitness contrasted with isolation exercises.

As a chiropractor or as an exercise professional, CrossFit is something that you have to be aware of and familiar with. It's important to know that the people who do it love it. If you ever bad mouth it or say anything negative about CrossFit to a CrossFit lover, you've basically lost them immediately. It is a lifestyle. People who get into it get into it big time. The CrossFit movement has created a <u>cult</u>-ure. It's almost like a family.

As you get into the Functional Fitness arena, I encourage you to research CrossFit. You're going to want to build a relationship with CrossFit gyms. They represent a big base of potential patients. You're going to want to get in there and understand how the trainers work, and you'll want to know the language. You can take some classes and get an idea of how they work. These boxes (hard for me to say, but that's what they call them), typically, will teach their clients mobility work. That's great if the client needs it. I've seen some boxes spend 10 to 15 minutes in the beginning of a session doing warm-up exercises. Then they usually have about a 20- to 25-minute workout, the Workout of the Day (WOD). That is followed by a cool-down session. This model has many great components included.

This sequence (warm-up, workout, cool down) is more in line with how we should be exercising and working out versus what is typically done when we go into a big box gym.

In a big box gym, a workout is usually a lighter repetition of the exercise that we're going to do, followed by a heavier version of the same thing. For example, if we're going to do chest workouts, we start with a lighter chest press and then do the heavy chest press. That doesn't activate a whole lot of stability. The weakness in that kind of workout is the client hasn't worked on much flexibility or stability prior to beginning their workout routine. The aim is isolation. The result may end in "dysfunctional fitness."

While I don't personally use CrossFit, because I do a lot of kettlebell training myself, I understand it, and I can respect when it's done well and done right.

A third style of Functional Fitness exercise that I want to mention is called "Movement Culture," which was developed by a guy named Ido Portal. Ido Portal, from Israel, is an interesting guy who is pretty outspoken. He does not keep it a secret that he feels that the bodybuilding era and the traditional way people are training for sports is very bad. He feels they're only training for aesthetics or just training for just specific activities, and they're not training for health and longevity. He often criticizes and critiques others. He calls them "poor movers."

This guy is pretty impressive, if you watch how he moves. He does a lot of things with gymnastic rings and a lot of "primal movements," which is a phrase that he uses quite a bit. He moves with animal-like grace, in crawling, rolling, and flipping. Ido makes the point that when someone is bodybuilding, they approaching it from the wrong angle. They get this aesthetically pleasing body, but they're very dysfunctional. They're strong in a single plane, but they're not healthy. This is a guy who is extremely flexible, very strong, shredded (low body fat with lean muscle mass), and in great physical condition. He's a really impressive guy. He's very opinionated, which might either turn you on or turn you off, but his approach to fitness is something that you should check out.

The three styles of Functional Fitness exercise that I've mentioned are ones you should be familiar with. I suggest that you check out YouTube videos and do some research to learn more about them. I did not cover every style or every practitioner. There are too many to cover in a limited space. When you learn the foundational ideas of Functional Movement and know the content of what we teach in MoveWell University, you'll be equipped to better evaluate and understand other exercise and fitness techniques you encounter.

When a new name pops up in functional fitness, you will know how to judge whether it's legitimate or just something being promoted that's not really based on any sort of evidence or science. As a Functional Movement practitioner, you need to be familiar with what's out there.

This is the conclusion of this chapter. We have much greater stuff to cover. If you got to this point without reading the previous chapters, you missed a lot of foundational material, so go back and start at the beginning. We'll see you in the next chapter.

CHAPTER 9

Why Not Functional Movement?

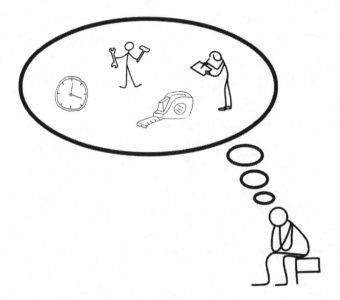

THIS CHAPTER DISCUSSES WHY PEOPLE ARE AFRAID TO incorporate functional movement into their practice.

There are two reasons chiropractors are not doing functional movement of any sort in their clinic. First, they're worried about the required space, time, staff, and training to deliver a quality experience for their patients. Second, they're worried that their patients won't see the value of functional movement.

These topics are briefly covered in our online training. The reasons above are kind of why I didn't do functional movement and exercise previously in my practice. I started with just adjusting for the first eight and a half years. Then I was introduced to a curve correction and postural corrective exercise, and that really intrigued me. It was like a new toy I got to figure out, and I was like, "Wow this is awesome!" I was starting to feel as though I was on autopilot in practice, and now I had this new component that I could offer to patients to further my results. So I implemented curve correction and postural corrective protocols, and after a few years of this combined approach, I realized there were still some missing pieces.

I started working out when I was 17 years old. I have enjoyed exercise and strength training for many years. Even with this background, when I became a chiropractor, I never incorporated any of the exercise approach into my clinical practice. So when I realized that I needed to add a functional exercise component to my practice, I didn't want this to be a generic model. I never wanted to simply have my patients hold a pink band and externally rotate their shoulder a thousand times, and then be satisfied that I was "incorporating exercise." Instead, if I was to pull the trigger and add corrective exercise into my practice (which I obviously did), I wanted to have these protocols directly carry over into preparing my patients for a safe and effective level of fitness. That's when it got really exciting for me. That was a big push for me to learn all this stuff.

With Tony (our exercise therapist at GSW) being in the fitness industry for so long, this is something he knows a lot about — how big of an industry this is. It's huge and it's growing, and I think, with all the information available online, it's just in everyone's face on social media, YouTube, etc. The exercise and fitness industry was something I started to see grow in the early 2000s, and it hasn't stopped. To me, it was a natural progression to integrate exercise and fitness into a chiropractic clinic.

From a weightloss standpoint, there are many chiropractic clinics that have moved into weightloss coaching, and the exercise component isn't being addressed. We're focusing on corrective exercise rehab, getting people moving and to the point where they can get into strength and power (you'd be surprised by how many patients are interested in that). That's something I think flows together very naturally. If you look at our content in MoveWell University and the way that the progressions work, you can see the change that occurs as a patient starts in the program. Maybe they've got an issue with their shoulder or their low back and they begin with isolated and simple movements to progress out of the painful stage. They will quickly evolve and grow into performing basic functional movement patterns. From there, they can very easily and naturally transition into strength training and power movements.

I've talked with some chiropractors who have their clinic inside of a gym or they actually own a gym. I know someone who owns a 15,000-square-foot gym and has chiropractic clinic inside it, and he owns it all. He has personal trainers to do the strength, power, and fitness components.

Tony adds, "The gym and chiropractic clinic model makes perfect sense to me, because when I was over in New York, we had a physical therapy clinic inside our gym. We had this contractor who would visit us every month or so and give talks and stuff. He was directly across the street, and that made a lot of sense to me that a healthcare provider would want to be part of the fitness environment."

There are pros and cons of having a gym with a chiropractic clinic inside. There are lots of pros. The only downside to having everything under one roof, including the personal training aspect, is that it would be challenging to get other personal trainers to refer to you, as they would see you as competition. Personally, I prefer the distinct role of the chiropractor and the fitness professional (personal trainer). The chiropractor is in charge of diagnosing and correcting injuries or underlying issues that are creating the movement dysfunction in the patient. The role of the fitness professional is to safely take the patient further into the strength and fitness aspect of exercise. We communicate this principle to our patients and do our best to motivate them to strive to set fitness goals, so physical exercise will become part of their lifestyle.

Let's talk about one of the biggest apparent obstacles when a chiropractor is contemplating adding corrective exercise into their practice: space. This is the biggest objection that I hear when chiropractors contact me to throw ideas around to see if they can add these protocols into their clinic. I cover this topic in our online webinar training. I have covered this in the MoveWell Podcast, and Tony and I have discussed this in video form. The great news is many of these protocols don't require a ton of space. I would say 90 percent of our protocols could be accomplished within a six-by-six-foot space. So the next variable is looking at how many patients you want to be able to see in a given hour.

Our clinic first started doing functional movement in a ten-by-ten-foot space. It can be done. Another major space-saving secret is using lacrosse balls and foam rollers. A lot of the mobility preparation work can be done with those. It is also important, as these are areas that enable you to anchor resistance bands. For example, in a 10-foot-by-10-foot space, you can anchor gear into the walls. If you have a little bit of a larger space, you can have freestanding equipment, which we have at our clinic. We have three Stroops "Performance Stations" that are freestanding, and resistance bands can be attached to them. We use the Stroops "Slastix" resistance band covered with a nylon sheath for safety and durability.

So you need to begin somewhere, and then you can scale up, as you either become creative with your existing space work or take on additional space. Many of the systems that we will cover in later chapters have enabled us to figure out many patients can be seen simultaneously, without sacrificing the quality of care. The moral of the story: As the volume grows, you're going to need a little bit more space, but you can get started in a small space.

In New Mexico, we started small when we didn't have the space and I was the associate doctor. If you're reading this and thinking, "I'd love to implement this stuff in practice, but I work for someone else and I don't call the shots," don't throw in the towel. The goal should be to present it to the clinic owner in the proper way and show how it can add value, add services, and add income by repurposing space in the practice that's not generating significant revenue. This is exactly what I did, and the clinic owner went for it. He was not someone who went for a lot of things, but he was sold.

Let me share what I did, to give you some perspective. Prior to converting to digital X-ray, we took full-spine X-rays on a 14x36, and we had a ton that needed to be stored. We had this room at the practice that was about 10 feet by 10 feet, and we had several of these huge steel X-ray racks that were stacked up to the ceiling and bolted to the walls.

So, I proposed the following to the clinic owner:

"What if I break all this down? And I'll pay for a monthly storage unit. And I'll handle moving all this out of the office. Then I'll fix up the walls and make this room look pretty. Can I take this room over? I will pay a percentage of what I bring to the clinic, and it will add value and add services for patients."

The clinic owner debated for a bit and then finally said ok. So my wife and I and a bunch of patients who owed me some favors went into the clinic, took the equipment down, and transported it to a storage space. We then had a space for traction and postural corrective exercise (mind you, I hadn't implemented the functional corrective exercise component yet, but it's the same principle). We fixed up all the walls. We built and purchased some equipment and we got rolling. We planned to start slow, but it took off very quickly. I also did weekly workshops and I invited all my existing patients. We introduced all these new things. We pitched patients on this and 50 percent of my practice, or more, converted and started using these new services, and it just blew up like crazy. Within three months, we were seeing over 150 patient visits per week on the exercise side of things.

In the next chapter, we are going to address another concern chiropractors have when implementing corrective exercise, the time aspect.

CHAPTER 10

The Time Objection

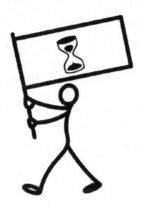

L ET'S CONTINUE THE CONVERSATION AS TO WHY CHIRO-
practors hesitate to add corrective exercise into their practice.
Another common objection that I hear is in regards to time.
There are a couple of things we will touch on regarding this. Perhaps currently, your practice model is focused solely on performing
adjustments, but you may be thinking, "How am I going to have
time to learn all this stuff and how to implement it?"

Well, you know we're always going to try to sneak in the plug
for MoveWell University. If you're a chiropractor reading this, take a
look at the MoveWell content (www.MoveWellUniversity.com and
register for one of our webinars) and you'll see that we did all of the
heavy lifting for you. We designed this program primarily to make
this implementation easy, concise, and time effective.

You already know all of the anatomy and how the body works,
but we cover a brief refresher just to bring you up to speed on how this
is going to play into understanding the functional component. What

the MoveWell content will add is critical organizational instruction, including flowcharts and documentation on how to organize your practice. We've made it so easy that you can finish all of the Move-Well content and have a really good understanding in just a week or two, with only an hour a day of study.

After we built MoveWell University, we tested it with our associate doctor, Dr. Zack. We had him go through all the content, and I think he got through it in about four days or so. First, he watched all of the video content, which only took about a day. Most of the videos are very short and to the point, except for a few more detailed, longer ones. Next, he practiced the protocols he wasn't familiar with, so he could understand and feel what a patient would be feeling. After that, he was confident enough to jump in and start implementing it clinically. Now, granted, he fast-tracked this process because he works in our clinic, but this will give you some idea of the timeframe needed to launch this process. We plan it out for a chiropractor who has little to no experience in corrective exercise, and we plan for this process to take up to four weeks. So for you, as a healthcare provider, you'll be able to learn the concepts very quickly.

A different concern might be that your patients are already in your office for twenty minutes or so to get adjusted, so how can you add more time? In our office, patients might be here for up to an hour to 90 minutes. We have a different model, but it is presented differently, and we run towards this possible objection with a patient right from the beginning. We present this as a positive thing, not a burden. This is a thorough type of clinical care, which is results driven. By investing the time that it takes to properly address your patient's problem, they are saving time and money in the long run and are, essentially, going to learn a curriculum of information they will be able to use for a lifetime.

I often use the quote: "Give a man a fish, feed him for a day, teach a man to fish, feed him for a lifetime." Then I will explain to a patient: "We firmly believe that for you to get healthy, our duty is to teach you how to fish."

Tony adds, "Back when I was a personal trainer, people would come in to see me for an hour-long session, two or three days a week. Some people did 90 minutes, while some people did two-a-days. If you get out in front of this thing and sell the value of it to patients early on, then 15 to 30 minutes more per visit isn't a problem. Fifteen minutes would be the bare minimum, though. If you're doing warm-up exercises, then spinal warm ups, then postural corrective exercise, then functional movement progressive exercises and if you are flying through it, it can be done in 15 minutes. But 15 minutes is the bare-bones minimum. On average, most of our patients are doing 30 minutes of this combination of exercise, and it is anything but a generic approach."

To add to what Tony shared, sometimes a patient arrives late to their appointment, and they're in a rush to get done. In that case, we quickly come up with a shortened exercise plan focusing on a select few protocols that are most important. The patient knocks those out and is out the door in 15 minutes. For the patients, that saves time. And I'm telling you, the patients who do functional movement (the right way, like we cover in this book) will quickly see the value in it. They're going to come back wanting more. They're going to have more questions and are going to want to do more progressions.

Honestly, you can provide even better care with a half hour or even 40 minutes. A major tip to make this successful is to make sure the communication aspect of your exercise department is dialed in. For example, when someone comes back and says they don't have enough time, the exercise therapists are the ones who hear about it. Addressing this objection is important, because if we are putting someone's care plan together, there is a clinical and a logistical component. We really don't want to diverge from the plan when the patient isn't giving us enough time to make progress. This will affect their results from a billing perspective. Whether it is dealing with health insurance or if it's an auto policy or workman's compensation, there is a business side to ensuring the patient is completing the billable services planned, in order to justify the staff, overhead, scheduling, etc. Our team knows how to handle these objections and "run towards the fire" to address these issues as they arise. If it is a situation that our staff feels that they cannot handle alone, they will immediately communicate this to the primary doctor, so we can handle the problem.

To further shamelessly plug MoveWell University, it will definitely save you time and money in this process, as you will not have to figure out these solutions on your own. This is whether you already have an exercise department or you are adding one from scratch. I am confident that our systems will be an improvement for almost any chiropractor.

Next, let's talk about the perceived obstacle of staffing and training an exercise department. If you don't have any staff working with you at this point, it can seem like this is going to be a huge problem. There are some doctors I've talked to who are implementing functional movement or have already done it and they only have one staff member. Besides scheduling, handling billing, and taking payments, they do everything. They're set up in a big open room and they're jumping in and jumping out of the room as needed. It can be done, but I would recommend investing in training an "exercise therapist" to help deliver those services, so you, the chiropractor, can focus on case management and adjustments.

As far as how we practice in our clinic, we practice the Gonstead method, and we have three individual changing rooms that lead into an adjusting room. This is with two adjusting rooms, so six changing rooms total. We're gowning and checking them with instrumentation each and every visit. With our layout, our patients can be adjusted in privacy (not out in the open), and then we have a whole separate open area for exercise. Now, you absolutely do not have to have this type of setup. I'm just sharing how we have built this to cater to our chiropractic methodology. I've heard of doctors who set up a T-bar wall, which provides some level of privacy with a four-foot wall. In this type of model, patients can be adjusted and then the doctor can jump back and forth and assist in the exercise area. Some prefer this style, while others prefer to hire more staff, so that the doctor assists in exercise if they are requested for a particular case. But in all reality, these systems are designed so the doctor designs and delegates the care, and the exercise therapists execute the delivery. Some of our MoveWell University doctors will help out, initially, with patient care in the exercise department. Once they are confident things are running smoothly, they will hire an additional exercise therapist and back out. This way, they can maintain a comfortable level of patient adjusting volume, and the additional staff in the exercise department can handle the increased exercise volume. That is the best model in my opinion, and again, these systems were designed to support this type of model.

And something that Tony and I have talked about in the past is that personal trainers are a really great resource if you're thinking about bringing somebody on board.

With MoveWell University, you can bring in a personal trainer and he or she is going to be familiar with many of the exercises. Conversely, it's also very simple for someone who isn't that familiar with functional movement and doesn't know a lot about anatomy. They can pick up the important parts fast using the training we provide in MoveWell University. It's not hard to implement at all. The reason that so many chiropractors don't implement functional movement or corrective exercise in their practice is because there's not a whole lot of information out there on how to do this in a turnkey fashion.

To give you some perspective on how we used to handle the staff training, I will share our past methods. When we first started implementing corrective exercise, we trained our staff by meeting late on Fridays and sometimes on Saturdays or Sundays. We'd all get together in our exercise room where I'd set up a camera and we'd start talking and going through exercises for two or three hours. Then I tried to use those videos as training for other staff. The problem was that it was two or three hours of unedited video. Tony can speak to this, as he was exposed to all of these old training videos.

Tony adds, "A lot of it was really very valuable. But as I was watching it, all I was thinking is that it's a good thing I'm a personal trainer because it allowed me to absorb it all. I was familiar with all of it, but to someone brand new to the idea, it would be really daunting."

We have since condensed it all down to the really important stuff. It's set up in a way that isn't nearly so difficult, and we use the MoveWell University membership site to train our staff. Our current staff still uses this program as a reference when they have a question, and when they come up with something that isn't in there, that is my cue that other members of our program may come across this question. So I will oftentimes add this information into the program.

It took us over six months to create MoveWell University, and our hard work and time spent creating this will benefit you even in the staff training component. If prior to reading this section, you were asking yourself how you're possibly going to take time out of your schedule to train new employees to add an exercise department, hopefully, this chapter has eased your mind.

On to the next...

CHAPTER 11

The "Nobody Will Care" Objection

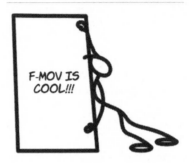

F-MOV IS COOL!!!

THIS NEXT CHAPTER DEALS WITH FEAR.

The fear is you're going to spend all this time developing this stuff and working out all of these details and your patients are going to see no value in it.

Tony explains, "I'm always talking about these parallels with personal training. I went to my martial arts instructor and he said, 'You should become a personal trainer.' So I went and got my certification. I got the National Academy of Sports Medicine (NASM) certification, because it was the hardest one and I'm that kind of guy. It took me three months to learn all the stuff. I show up for my first day and I started to worry if I would get clients or not. And I had a lot of same feelings when Dr. Todd developed MoveWell. I was worried if we could make it happen, but sure enough, we did."

Before Tony became a part of our clinic staff, we had systems, but we didn't have the best systems. We developed our initial protocols and procedures before he came in. It took us a lot of time to put them together.

Initially when our staff ran through the exercises with our patients, they weren't super excited about doing them. As a result, they weren't motivating our patients. The motivation is crucial to adding value to the practice of corrective exercise and functional movement.

What we needed and what you need is excited staff. Excited staff will ignite excitement within your patients and the patients, in turn, will see the value in the program.

Tony adds, "This is a similar approach as with personal training. You have to 're-sell' personal training every single time. You don't want to take that patient or client for granted, and you don't want to assume that they are 100 percent stoked and on board, when maybe it's going to take you getting them there every single time."

My original mentor in chiropractic told me, "You're only as good as your last adjustment." So that means you can work miracles for your patient for 20 visits in a row, but on visit 21, if you don't engage with the patient in the right way, the patient loses some of their enthusiasm for chiropractic care and decides not to come back.

One of the things that is important to look for in hiring somebody, even if they're not a personal trainer, is hiring someone who is excited about exercise and movement. Their excitement is going to be noticeable when they talk about the functional movement protocols. They will be teaching with enthusiasm. Contrast this with a person who doesn't like working out. They won't be able to get the patient excited about care.

Tony explains, "When I was interviewed for this job, I wasn't quite sure why I was being asked what I did for exercise or activities and stuff. But now I realize it was because you want people in your clinic who are genuinely interested in and appreciate movement, fitness, and exercise."

If you can hire an experienced and competent fitness professional, like a personal trainer, that's great. But there's a caution. Insurance contracts in some states require that clinical staff who provide support services to covered providers (the chiropractor) have particular certifications and are a Certified Medical Assistant (CMA), Registered Medical Assistant (RMA), or a Certified Nursing Assistant

(CNA). A personal trainer certification by itself does not generally qualify under these contracts.

If you are working under such an insurance contract and you are hiring one person, you need to hire a person who will comply with the contract requirements. If you have two or more people in your exercise department, you could hire someone with a CMA, RMA, or CNA certification and hire an enthusiastic trainer as one of your staff. The trainer can work with patients under the supervision of the certified staff member, engage your patients, and be a resource for the team.

Personal trainers tend to try to get other people around them interested in health and fitness. So even if you have three people in the exercise department and only one of them is a personal trainer, the trainer is going to get the other two excited about the stuff you are doing at the clinic. If they're around the trainer all day long, it's going to rub off on them. If the enthusiasm for exercise and fitness doesn't infect the other members of the exercise staff, it's going to be pretty apparent they're not a great fit for the job. Hopefully, you can screen the people who aren't enthusiastic about fitness before you hire them. But even if you can't, they will disqualify themselves for the job by their lack of conviction.

Getting back to how we got started. We didn't have people who were excited about fitness and movement. We didn't have staff who knew how to organize the protocols.

We had many protocols to choose from, and we were experimenting with different approaches, trying to decide what was the best way and the best time to introduce exercise and movement to the patient. We didn't have a system in place to track patient history and progress. Sure, our patient management and billing system let us keep track of which treatment codes were being done at each visit, but the exercise staff couldn't see the big picture of the progression of the patient.

And from the patient's standpoint, they didn't see where they were going in a clear, systematic way. We didn't present to the patient a clear step-by-step process.

Looking for a solution to this problem led us to the belt system. Tony came up with the idea of "The Belt System of Functional Movement." Part of the belt system was explaining to a patient just doing the same exercises over and over wasn't enough to help them achieve improvement in their ability to move with better competency. Going through a progression of protocols was what was going to help them the most.

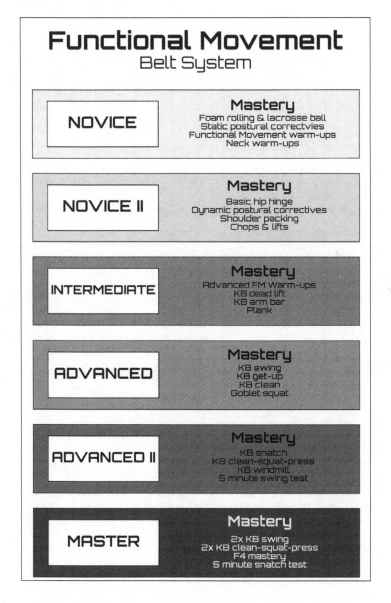

It's not just, "Ok, here's the lacrosse ball. Roll around on this." There's this whole progression of anywhere between six to 15 different exercises.

Ideally, what we're doing is trying to take our patients and demonstrate the importance of lifetime spinal and functional health. That's best for them and their total well-being. We don't seek to make them a "three times a week forever" patient. Instead, we aim to inspire our patients to put in the work and dedication required, in order to correct and stabilize the cause of their problem. Once stabile, they can then incorporate the principles we have taught them into their daily or weekly activities. What does that mean? We teach our patients how to begin their day with a morning routine that includes their spinal rehabilitation exercises. And we stress the importance of adopting a weekly functional exercise regimen that can be executed long-term. And do you want to know the really cool part about this? Patients welcome this. They want this, and they follow it, as long as there are systems in place to hold them accountable.

As a patient progresses in treatment, we back off with their recommended frequency of care. We see the patient less frequently, but provide more services and spend more time per visit, therefore increasing the value to the patient. We empower the patient with resources to show them what they can do at home, between appointments.

What type of feedback do we get? They love this!

As a result, our patients are more likely to refer, and they're more likely to stick with this approach in the long term. When you follow these systems, this will increase your patient count. You will get busy so quickly with this approach that you will want your ongoing (supportive care) patients to be seen less frequently, so you can make room for all of the newer people coming in.

The last thing that I want to mention about this belt system is what you say to a patient who asks you, "Well, can I just do this stuff at home?" We tell the patient that the reason we make these resources available to them is so that they can see where they're going with the exercise program, and, absolutely, they need to be doing these things at home. And as they do them at home, each time they come to the clinic for a visit, we're going to give them progressions and things to work on for continued improvement. They will have access to an online "exercise library" to help them correctly perform their prescribed protocols. We invite them to check out the ones that aren't prescribed to them if they'd like but realize that those may not be appropriate for them yet.

We remind them that it is in their best interest to follow our guidance so they achieve the best results. We let them know that on each one of their visits, we will review their prescribed home care exercises to check in and see how they are doing. We will re-assess their movement competency and make sure they understand all of the little cues in the exercises they've been doing. Either they will stay at that level until they improve, or we will progress them to the next level.

We talked about fear at the beginning of this chapter:

The fear of objections from a patient.

The fear that this program might have no value for patients.

We created an online membership site our patients gain access to, and they use this as a resource as they progress through the program. This online portal is the 12-Week Transformation, and it eliminates the reasons for these fears. Further, it serves to demonstrate the comprehensive value of this program to our patients.

We've done the work to make this program available to doctors and their patients. We have cloned the entire 12-Week Transformation, which is part of our MoveWell University doctor training program. So, again, you have the ability to gain access to a clone of this program, which can be further customized to your office and your practice style. The 12-Week Transformation contains a comprehensive exercise library that is accessible by your patients. It already contains close to 80 patient of the education videos that are drip-fed over the 12-week period. You can add or delete any of the videos based on your personal preferences and style of patient care. This is a curriculum for overall health, including spine and posture care, and functional movement. It even touches on strength and power, as we go through a kettlebell section with StrongFirst Master Instructor, Zar Horton.

Touching on how we began this chapter, where we mentioned the fear of your patient not seeing the value in this program, I hope you feel confident that we have successfully taken that objection and twisted it, crushed it, and threw it in the trash. As we review all of the bells and whistles within our exercise program, it should be apparent that these systems are solid. We have helped replicate these systems in chiropractic clinics all across the country, and the feedback that we have received from these doctors is awesome.

The goal of this chapter was to make a compelling case that you too, can have these systems in place. We've given you a solution for excitement and the insight of why you need to learn this, how you can do this, and why this is such an amazing opportunity to add a department like this into your practice. Are you excited yet?

The next chapter talks about implementing functional movement.

CHAPTER 12

Implementation

N THIS CHAPTER, WE WILL BE DISCUSSING ALL OF THE moving parts involved in implementation.

If you're just getting started with this stuff, you don't need a lot of equipment. The basic equipment is very easy to acquire and very inexpensive. It includes some lacrosse balls, foam rollers, and resistance bands with various attachments. With these alone, you can do a large number of the protocols that we go over in Move-Well University. From this starter set, you can just keep building and keep adding as you get more patients participating in the functional movement exercises.

Stepping back for a minute, in order to have a well-rounded corrective exercise department, you will need to have protocols in place that address mobility/flexibility, patterning/motor control, and strength/power.

For the mobility component, first we have a variety of trigger point and muscle work tools and protocols that we teach our patients. We primarily use a theracane trigger point tool, lacrosse balls, and foam rollers. You can do a lot with these basic pieces of equipment.

The equipment required for most of the patterning and motor control protocols is as simple as resistance bands and PVC pipes. I like the Stroops 'Slastix' bands, as they are covered with a vinyl sheath, and if they break (all resistance bands will eventually break), your patient will not be injured.

To briefly touch on the concept of a "motor control" exercise, let me break it down. Once a patient has regained or demonstrated that they have mobility and flexibility in their soft tissue and joints, let's say in a forward-bending toe-touch pattern, this isn't always enough for them to be able to regain this necessary functional movement pattern. They may have a "motor control" problem, which is often exactly the case. This means that they lack the neural coordination and support to complete the movement functionally. In the case of the toe-touch example, this will occur when the patient lacks spine stability. When they bend forward to touch their toes, and if they do not possess the proper spinal stability from their core and deep musculature, the brain goes into protect mode and it applies a "braking" mechanism to the posterior chain muscles, the hamstrings, and the low back. So when the patient bends forward, even though they have acceptable flexibility in the low back and hamstrings, as soon as they attempt to execute a weight-bearing forward-bending toe touch, things tighten up and they struggle to complete the movement. The brain is creating this stiffness as a protective mechanism. So how do you correct this? There are specific protocols that will retrain the stability aspect as the patient enjoys the forward flexion movement. This is done in repetition, and this is one of the initial steps in re-training a functional movement pattern that has been lost. Are you still with me? Cool. Let's continue.

PVC pipes are an inexpensive and effective tool for teaching your patient how to maintain a neutral spine, especially when they're learning how to properly hip hinge. The pipes are also a great aid used in shoulder mobility drills as well as ankle mobility exercises (ankle stick drill).

Some of the stability exercises don't require any equipment other than a floor mat or something that will let a patient get down on the floor and be comfortable. For example, a really simple type of exercise that everyone should be doing involves coaching the proper breathing pattern. Breathing is a coordinated functional movement exercise. Another foundational exercise that we really like to use, especially in people who have a rotary stability problem, is the body roll, where a patient lays on the ground and practices rolling from supine to prone and then prone to supine by primarily using their core without momentum from the extremities. If you have never tried body rolling, it is harder than you think, and this is a great exercise *and* an assessment, as it can expose huge asymmetries that are hiding in other activities. These two movements do not require any equipment other than a mat, and they're invaluable.

The message is to get the ball rolling, you don't need a lot of equipment. So don't let equipment requirements be something that scares you away. You don't need a lot of it.

We use a lot of Stroops equipment in our clinic. Stroops is a supplier of premium fitness equipment. We use Stroops because it's high quality and it looks classy for something that's fairly simple. You take a band and you cover it with a vinyl sleeve. Not only does it look cooler, but it's also safer. If it snaps, it won't injure someone. Part of what makes your exercise department attractive is having a unique look to what you're doing. Make the equipment something that's a little different than what patients would see in a gym or buy on their own. Most people don't know about Stroops. They even have special packages that they put together for our MoveWell University members.

Moving on. Let's talk about space planning. I know some of this overlaps of what we talked about in our previous chapters where we talked about the space concern. If you're just starting exercise — let's say you've repurposed some space — you might start in a smaller space and then figure out how you're going to scale and figure out your space needs based on how many patients you're going to see per hour and how many exercise staff members you have.

We do a lot of different things in our functional movement department space. Depending on what's going on with your clinic, you can do more than just functional movement exercises in a room. I don't think that you need to have a special area where only functional movement exercises are done. We do our assessments in this area as well as our "Day Four" procedures with the patient there. Day Four is where we onboard our patients with the 12-Week Transformation, go over their home care protocols, and talk about goal-setting. We also do our manual therapy in our functional movement area, so if that is something you do in your clinic, you can share the space. I don't want you to think you necessarily have to have separate rooms or a whole new room just for functional movement.

In some cases, we've had doctors who have completely moved equipment from one larger room to another room just so that the area that is being designated for exercise is easier to upscale in the future, as the volume demands call for it. This is something to consider as you get started. Expect it to grow and expect it to blow up, because this can grow quickly. If you start with solid systems and cover all the key points that we're covering in this book, it's going to work. So if you can, plan it to be scalable.

Now we'll deal with designing assessment and exercise protocols. It's important to understand what other assessments exist in this space. The primary screening is called the Functional Movement Screen (FMS) and the most popular assessment out there is the Selective Functional Movement Assessment (SFMA).

Tony explains, "When we were developing the MoveWell 3 screening, even as a very experienced exercise person with really good understanding of anatomy, it took me three or four months to really get comfortable applying the SFMA. It is a great assessment tool. It is very thorough and takes about half an hour. You have to sit back and ask yourself, as a healthcare practitioner, 'What do I really need?'

Dr. Todd and I talked a lot about this 90 percent thing. We're trying to capture 90 percent of the dysfunctions that you're going to see, and do it in a timely fashion. This is why we created the MoveWell 3. It can be performed in under seven minutes, and it gives us a ton of information to get started with a patient."

If you're not opposed to continuing education, we recommend learning the FMS and the SFMA. It's a really good base to fall back on and to understand, as the clinician. You don't have to learn both in order to implement the MoveWell 3, but I would say, if you can do it, you should.

We designed the MoveWell 3 system based on what we commonly see in practice and how this flows smoothly with our other clinical interventions. Initially, our approach was, "Let's pull the best from everything. Let's pull some things out that we want to test that are not included in the screening and the assessment, and let's build this thing called the MoveWell 3." By the time we were done, we found that it is much quicker for us to use the MoveWell 3 than it is to do a full blown SFMA on everyone.

The SFMA is a wonderful assessment. But, for example, we did not want to spend time testing the patient's vestibular system. It is not something we deal with much at the clinic, especially if we've already spotted that they have a shoulder, thoracic, and cervical dysfunction. We're going to have so much to work on, the odds are we will never get to deal with the vestibular system, so the time spent on that part of the assessment would be of little value to us and of little value to the patient.

Side note: If we are concerned about a vestibular issue, we will detect this in our initial day-one examination and address accordingly.

It doesn't make sense to assess aspects of the patient's movement that we're not going to deal with or we are not set up to handle. How we've done this clinically is we say, "We're going to start at a certain level. If we get to a stopping point or if we see certain red flags along the way, we need to factor that into our examination of the patient."

For example, if you're taking a patient through a single-leg stance exercise, or perhaps a position in tall kneeling (anything that separates left and right side of the body) and the patient starts getting dizzy and loses balance, we may decide to test their balance. We have a conversation and, from there, decide what to do. Do we refer them out to a therapist, for example, who specializes in vestibular training? Vestibular training is not something that we really want to do or specialize in.

You may think that you want to design the most in-depth testing protocols ever. By the time you're done, it's 90 minutes long. Keep in mind this is something that you're going to have to teach to your employees. And every time a new person comes on, you're going to have to teach them. Contrast that with the MoveWell 3. It is an assessment that you can initially teach your staff in an afternoon. They'll need to practice it a little bit, sure, but it's not hard to pick it up and it won't take as long to teach and to learn as a more complicated assessment.

In designing the assessment, we found that we needed a scoring system — an objective number, a score — so that you can say, "You were a 15 two weeks ago, now you are 17." It is important that we are able to retest in order to see improvement. Nine times out of 10, patients will ask how they did, and when you can tell the patient "you used to be a 15, and now you are a 17," they tend to get really excited about that. People want to feel like they're making progress. Having these protocols with a numerical value that you can use for comparison is really powerful.

Another reason that the assessment is so important is because the assessment is a justification of the value of the treatment services you're going to provide. For example, your assessment might encompass a range of motion on multiple joints or a range of motion that you can extrapolate from certain movement patterns. Perhaps you have the patient do a reaching pattern, and from that you can get a pretty accurate idea of what their shoulder range of motion is, their flexion, and internal and external rotation. You document that. Perhaps the results suggest that you found a key issue, so you dive in a little further and do some special tests after the first assessment. One of the reasons that you need the assessment and the documentation is because if you are billing health insurance for this, you need to have a documented assessment to show that you found a problem in order to justify the care that you then rendered. Once you've taken the patient through a care plan, you re-do the assessment and now you have an objective way of measuring whether it changed or it stayed the same.

We have condensed the MoveWell 3 assessment to 50 or 60 of the most important items. There are easily hundreds of items that you could include in an assessment. You could probably design a few assessments yourself, if you wanted to. Some systems boast about how many different exercises they have the patient do as part of their assessment. The fact is that extraneous exercises as part of the assessment just add more layers of confusion for your department, for your doctors and for the patient. And remember, you're going to have to teach all this stuff to your functional movement team. So just keep it simple.

We have identified a group of kettlebell exercises that encompass every important functional movement out there. We call it the Functional Four. The patient should not initially do these with a personal trainer, at a gym, or working out on their own, but they need to do them in front of your highly trained staff AFTER they have demonstrated the appropriate mobility and stability, to ensure that they are safe to proceed.

The functional four include:

1. THE DEADLIFT PATTERN: here we teach how to hip hinge and safely deadlift.
2. THE KETTLEBELL SWING: reinforcing the hip hinge and loading the posterior chain.
3. THE KETTLEBELL GOBLET SQUAT: patterning the triple flexion vertical descent movement.
4. THE KETTLEBELL GETUP: seven specific steps on the way up and back down.

Regarding the Getup, this is complicated, but it's probably one of the more fun exercises to learn because it's so different. The kettlebell get up serves as an assessment as well as an exercise. It is comprised of seven different movements on the way up and on the way back down. There are things you can identify in the get up to assess what movement deficiencies might be hiding.

I need to add an important note about the Dynamic Kettlebell Swing. If you go to most gyms and watch people perform kettlebell swings, oftentimes they have not been taught all that well. Common errors include pulling the bell up super high or squatting while they swing instead of hip hinging. There are all kinds of errors that a person might do in a swing. When the swing is done properly, it is a functional exercise to reinforce healthy patterns.

We picked these four because they are the four best exercises for reinforcing healthy patterns and improving functional movement. I don't think there's anything better that encompasses these fundamental, primal, full-body movement patterns.

THE FUNCTIONAL FOUR (EXERCISES) ▲

What is the Functional Four? >

● Deadlift >

● Swing >

● Goblet Squat >

● Get-Up >

So as a patient becomes more advanced with the corrective exercise basics, and they step up to the plate to begin learning the Functional Four, this gives you a new, more advanced version of a screening and movement assessment. If they're struggling on certain steps in these four kettlebell exercises, you can then back up and plug in correctives to fix these identified deficiencies.

An important point: Our goal is to get every single patient to do a hip hinge and a deadlift. We have even had cases in which a patient has a full-spine fusion and their movement is very limited and we are able to teach them how to perform some level of a deadlift, even if it's four inches of movement onto an elevated platform. We want them to understand how to hip hinge and how to do it supporting a load, even if it's a light load. One of the great things about the deadlift is it is very modifiable. Even an elderly patient, or someone who has a lot of movement issues, can do at least partial range of motion, and it's really valuable in their everyday life.

That sums it up for our implementation section. In the next chapter, we're going to start talking about the importance of documentation and the different types.

CHAPTER 13

Documentation

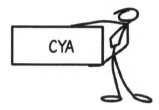

I N THIS CHAPTER, WE ARE GOING TO DISCUSS THE DOCU-mentation process involved with implementing corrective exercise and functional movement. Many clinicians are afraid of the documentation process. The first thing we will discuss regarding documentation is tracking. Tracking means your patients are going to come back into your exercise area, wherever that is in your clinic, and track their progress. There's a lot of stuff you will track, but one thing that is important is to track what exercises they are doing each day and how much time they spend completing those exercises. In our functional movement department, we have an entire card designated just for a patient's functional movement progress, as well as what is recommended for them as they continue their appointments. Sometimes we have up to six people back in our functional movement department and they're all doing different things. You have to make sure your staff knows what the patients are supposed to be doing and you're keeping track of the specific exercises and the amount of time they're spending for billing purposes.

If you're working with insurance, there are specific compliance guidelines that will require a certain qualified staff member to work with them so you can satisfy those requirements. In most states, with self-pay patients, there are no guidelines for staff certification requirements or time spent, but it's important to check with your state, since some may have special rules. Again, for billing purposes, it's important to keep track of how much time someone is spending in each different classification of exercise. Also, tracking their exercise time is important in order to ensure the patient isn't exercising too long. From a business standpoint, you may be spending extra time with a patient who hasn't paid for those services.

Tracking also plays a key role in illustrating a patient's progress. It's helpful to show a patient how they're doing to keep them motivated. This helps keep them excited about what they're doing. It really means a lot to people when you pull out their exercise card and they see all of the progress they've made. You can even say to them, "Hey, remember when you couldn't hip hinge? It took us a couple of weeks to get that down and now you're doing kettlebell deadlifts. You should be proud of yourself."

People get really excited when they can see the documentation showing all of the progress that they've made.

There are two main documents that we have for tracking purposes. One is the master document, which is our travel card that moves with the patient all around the clinic from the beginning to the end of their appointment. And the second one is our exercise card that remains in the exercise department. We perfected the travel card over time, with over 20 revisions. There are many purposes to the travel card. One of the main purposes is each department can see what every other department is doing or have done that day, which is super important. As the doctor, you're busy and your staff is doing an awesome job directing the flow of patients. So let's say you see a patient and you would like to look up something about their appointments. In just seconds, you can see that they've already done their exercises, and more specifically, you can see how long they spent on them.

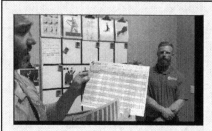

The Exercise Card
Efficient & Compliant

Your staff's ability to track a patient's progression form visit to visit is crucial. This document works hand in hand with our dry erase board system which, like every part of MoveWell University, we cover in detailed video training.

The Travel Card
The Systems Begin Here

Paper? You are still using paper?
Yes...and here is what we have found...

As digitally driven as a clinic can be, we have found determined that the level of moving parts in a clinic that integrates corrective exercise, a travel card is a must.

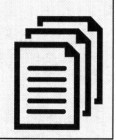

Tony adds: "Similarly, in the functional movement department, they are able to see if the patient has seen the doctor yet. Frequently, a patient will ask the exercise staff a question that really should be directed to Dr. Todd. In that case, the exercise therapist can acknowledge their question and tell them to ask Dr. Todd, knowing that they will see him next. The main purpose of tracking is to create communication between the staff and the patient."

Another way we use tracking to communicate between staff is through instant messenger. Each staff computer has an instant messenger window open, where we can communicate through a group chat or an individual chat, if needed. I have a scribe in my adjustment room, which is really beneficial and has made my life a lot easier. It helps to have a scribe doing documentation and running things throughout the clinic. And oftentimes, other departments will send my scribe a direct message through instant messenger to verify where I'm at with each patient.

After the patient has completed their services in each department, the travel card then goes to the front desk. The front desk staff uses the travel card to enter the number of units each patient should be billed for that day. Then, their travel card is audited and checked against the charges in our system before it gets billed, to make sure it's all consistent. We double-check to make sure we're hitting certain time markers as planned and it's all fitting together perfectly.

Another purpose of the travel card is maintaining compliant notes and records. We use the travel card to help compile our notes for the patient for the day. The travel card allows us to keep track of the category of exercises that a patient completes during each visit.

The exercise card helps us organize the specific protocols that are prescribed to the needs of the patient. Patients have warm-up exercises that may be different from one another, depending on their situation. They also have certain types of corrective exercises for their posture. In addition, they will have a specific set of functional movement progressive exercises based on their movement deficiencies and unique clinical findings.

Our exercise card is set up in such a way that it's very easy and fast to take in information at the end of the shift and get it right into the patient's electronic health record in the computer. It's important to separate all the different therapies and services out for billing purposes. For example, we have to know how many minutes are going to count towards a therapeutic exercise and how many are going towards a therapeutic activity. There's a list of parameters pertaining to different types of exercise that would make them fall into one category or the other. You will have to understand that as well.

We hired a compliance coach who observed in our clinic for several months. He looked at what we had in place and told us what was good and what needed improvement. He provided a ton of value and some great ideas for what we needed to fix and what parameters to follow. However, he didn't give us the forms or other turnkey materials. Instead, we would spend dozens of hours designing a document and then take it to him and he would provide ideas and feedback of what to change or add. The moral of the story is that you need to run an exercise department in a compliant fashion. We went above and beyond to make sure we had one of the top compliance guys on our team to ensure that we had everything in line.

Compliant notes have a series of parameters that must be met. If there is a time code, you need to record the time that the patient engages per service. This would apply to procedures such as therapeutic exercise, therapeutic activities, manual therapy, and the physical performance test. Any sort of time-sensitive processes or procedures must be timed per service. Then you have to add up the total time underneath each individual timed code. We have buttons in our electronic health records system where you hit a button that says "time pre-service" or "total time." It's all added up and we make sure that those numbers jive to what we have on our exercise form. From there, you have to make sure you have the appropriate diagnoses to support the procedure code.

So this is originally set up by our doctors, but our staff is awesome and they understand the process and know how to catch something that's missing. They alert us before it's billed out and possibly denied by the insurance company. We have several checks and balances, so if a patient is doing a manual therapy service, for example, it has its own diagnosis code. If the doctor performed an extremity adjustment that same visit, in order for that to be a billable service, the extremity adjustment and the manual therapy have to be in different regions of the body. All those details have to be outlined and your team must be trained to make sure the billing team, front office, and the exercise staff are all on the same page.

Let's talk about the patient self-tracking concept for the work that they do outside of the office. We previously touched on what we call our Day Four, or the Exercise Orientation visit. On this day we introduce the different moving pieces in this corrective care model, including the exercise department and the concepts behind functional movement. We give the patient their 12-Week Transformation journal that they're going to take home with them. And guess what we have in there? We have all of these great charts for tracking their home care (exercise, stretching, traction, etc.) Everyone is given clearly defined work to do at home. And from day one, they're hearing the importance of home care and tracking their performance. If they're not tracking their work at home, there's a good chance that they're not doing it. If you help them understand the importance of tracking their progress from the beginning, they will implement this into their home care.

It's critical that all of the staff, the doctors, exercise therapists, and even the front office are regularly asking the patients how their home care is going and if they have any questions about it. Early on, we also remind them that this exercise journal should follow them into the clinic every time they come for an appointment. And guess what, people don't follow directions. So we tell them to bring it in and then they say that they "forgot it." Then we "punish them" by writing on a sticky note instead and telling them to go copy these notes into their journal when they get home. Since they just created an additional step because they failed to bring their journal in, they are less likely to forget next time. To make this work, you have to be consistent with the message. If you just say that one time and then you allow three or four visits to go by without using the journal, they're going to deviate back to forgetting about their booklet, not using it to write down new protocols or questions that will arise when they are performing their exercises at home. They are taught to reference the exercise library inside of the 12-Week Transformation. We identify the names of the specific exercises that they should be working on that week, and they have a resource to access these video protocols. It works great.

Once they're using the journal consistently, they can't say they weren't given good guidance or didn't have a chance to ask questions. Our team reminds them, "If you remember, that's why we want you to bring your journal with you so you can get the most value out of this. We want you to do awesome with this program. I'm sure that's what you are looking for as well, right?"

This concludes the documentation section and gives you a blueprint for what you have to make sure you have covered when you set up your exercise department. And besides that, I think we're ready to move on to the next section, which is communication. So get ready. This one helps bring it all together.

CHAPTER 14

Communication

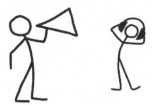

T HIS CHAPTER DISCUSSES COMMUNICATION. THREE main points include the value for the patient between the staff and then with the doctor, and we're going to talk a little bit about things we've learned along the way.

A lot of this information regarding communication overlaps with other sections, but we are addressing it from different angles so you understand the importance. So first let's discuss communication with the patient and the value in it. The vast amount of communication we initially do with a patient when they start the exercise program is on Day Four. We call that visit the functional movement orientation day, or Exercise Orientation.

The Exercise Orientation, as we touched on in an earlier segment, immediately introduces our journal as part of the communication process. Literally, the minute they come in, I sit them down and we talk about their 12-Week Transformation booklet. This booklet becomes a tool for communication between the functional movement department and the patient. The way to be most effective with your client or athlete, when you're starting off with them, is by setting goals.

This is a 12-week process and how we see our patients clinically. So we set 12 goals. So we would tell you to make sure you write down and set goals of your patient. Write three short-term goals right there. When a patient has objections to their treatment plan, we will flip back to their booklet and show them their goals and walk them through our plan of treatment again.

Objections are something we teach to our team because we use MoveWell University as a team training, and we have a whole section about the top nine objections patients have. A lot of the stuff you may hear in an exercise department can be used. This is really important. Your functional movement staff has to really get this stuff and get the communication because they spend more time with the patients than the chiropractor does on most visits. Sometimes, the functional movement staff will have 45 minutes with a patient and there's a lot of communication that goes on in that time. Adding an exercise department has improved retention and, especially, retention through the process. Then I would say retention afterwards for some level of wellness or follow-up care because they get it. They see how invested we are in someone's health that they understand this is something that they need to incorporate in their life forever. They know they're not going to find it anywhere else in any of the chiropractic clinics, so I'll tell you honestly, it happens every once in a while. The patient who jumped ship goes to another chiropractor.

Overcoming Objections

Hear what they aren't saying...

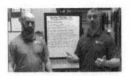

Objection #1: "I'm Too Busy"

Too busy for your health? No way!

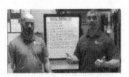

Objection #2: "I'm Feeling Great!"

But is health how you LOOk or how you FEEL? I didn't think so...

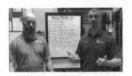

Objection #3: "I Can't Afford Care..."

But can you afford a Starbucks?

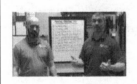

Objection #4: "But My Other Chiro Charged Me xxx"

You get what you paid for...

The Top 9 Objections & How to Handle Them – Part of the MoveWell University Membership site: www.MoveWellUniversity.com

Another thing is making sure you're casting your net of marketing and everything to the demographic you really want to bring in, which, in my opinion, are some of the most favored patients anyway, because they are usually fitness people who already understand health. It's just at this point, for me, I'm ready to work smarter and really market our target demographic. Ultimately, all this communication builds tremendous value for the patient, so they can visualize themselves going through the program and they understand what to expect and how we talk about it.

When doing the Exercise Orientation, we train our team to tell patients pretty much four things. The first thing is to review what the patient did last time and what they're going to do today. And then tell them at the end what they did today and then what they're going to do next time.

Keep in mind, you know people are very busy. Everyone has a lot of other commitments. And you at your clinic, you're always going to be vying for people's time, especially if they're coming in for a 45-minute visit. It's important to re-establish value just like we've talked about.

Communication between the staff is very important. We have a large team of people jammed under one roof to work together as a fully functional yet dysfunctional family. I can't tell you that it's perfect all the time, because it's never going to be perfect in any business. We are human beings, but we can improve our imperfections by having great communication. As an employer, you get some people who really want to take their work seriously and have stellar communication. And you have others who might be dealing with stuff in their personal life that they bring into the workplace that they shouldn't. And sometimes it blows up into a problem. Ultimately, what we are talking about is not necessarily counseling for your staff as far as how to get along, but it's talking about how to prevent those issues from a procedural standpoint to begin with. You need really solid procedures and communication processes, so you don't add that to all the other variables that are hard to predict or control and kind of come with the territory of just being human.

Using our staff system, let's say that you're setting up patients for the day. We use a dry erase board system to map everything out with the information on the patient's exercise card. And of this information comes from our computer system where we have everyone and their schedule listed. Also, pertinent information is copied over to the patient's exercise card from the doctor's recommendations. And hopefully, we only do that each time we have to get a new exercise card. It's better just to do it all at once.

An important thing to train your staff on is if you have someone who's more seasoned and someone who is less seasoned. Let's say that less seasoned person is instructing someone on an exercise and maybe the person is not doing it correctly and that less seasoned person doesn't catch it and they don't make a correction. The more seasoned employee would then step in and say, "I see you working on X, Y, or Z. Let me show you a couple of details about that, so you're not showing them that what they're doing is wrong and this is right way. You're showing them a slightly different way of doing it.

Communication is important for keeping the doctor in the loop along with the rest of the team, especially when it involves the patient's functional movement and where they stand. It's important that the doctor stays up to date with which exercises they've mastered and which exercises they're still learning and which exercises are coming up next. The way our computer system is set up, you can click on a patient and you can see how the patient is doing in terms of the belt system. You can see not only what belt level the patient is currently at, but every protocol they've done since they've started at the clinic. We set it up this way to make it easier on ourselves, and we're sharing this all with you so you don't have to go through the whole learning process like we did. Over time, we have added different codes. For instance, we've narrowed it down now where if there was a surgical dysfunction for example, we call this D-1, or dysfunction one. The exercise staff can just type it in chat or in the system and say we're going to need D-1 white belt level. And I immediately know exactly what that means based on this belt system card, and everything is very streamlined and simplified. And if there's multiple different areas we can have a D-1, D-4, and D-7, we will list it in order of priority. And then they know, immediately, to look at all the white belt protocols. Let's start with the first priority dysfunction and go through that. Once they evolve past that, they get into the functional movement system master list. And then after they've cleared that out, we see if there anything left over for them to do. Sometimes, there is, and they finish that up. Boom. Now they're done with white belt. They graduate and then get a yellow belt. Then the patient gets rewarded and it's a celebration, like, "Hey, you've you finished everything in white belt and you're now going into the yellow belt. Awesome. Great work. Great job." And then we give them a white belt. They have that. And then our team will send a message on our group instant messenger to say, "Hey, John just went up to the yellow belt today. Make sure you congratulate him." And then the whole team makes it the celebration fun.

The last thing to touch on, and the reason communication is so important, is your exercise staff has to be comfortable if they feel some sort of hesitation from a patient to bring it to the doctor's attention. If the patient seems frustrated, like they don't want to be there, and it seems like they're trying to rush through something, the doctor needs to be able to address that. If a patient is showing these signs, you have to decode their nonverbal communication to understand what they are saying. In this situation, very little is being said through verbal communication. It's all body language. This is where a stellar exercise staff comes into play. For instance, if a patient is frustrated while doing their functional movements, an exercise staff member could privately say, "Hey, John it seems like maybe this exercise is a little bit frustrating for you. Now, is it that you are you are just wondering how much longer it will take to do exercise? Or are you looking to progress? Is there something we can do to improve this for you?" Calling the patient out and addressing the situation is may seem awkward, but it's really not that awkward. Addressing the situation earns the patient's respect, because the patient realizes the exercise staff picked up on the nonverbal messages.

I think we pretty much wrapped it up with communication. The next part that we're going we're to get into is departmentalizing.

CHAPTER 15

Departmentalizing

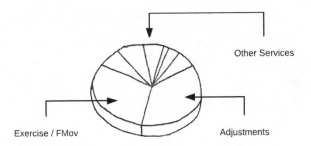

Other Services

Exercise / FMov

Adjustments

D
EPARTMENTALIZING YOUR PRACTICE, WHICH IS NOT
to be confused with departmentalization, has been a key
aspect of my business model at GSW.

When I first began learning about Chiropractic BioPhysics and corrective care with traction, I was aware of a chiropractic clinic that was medically integrated, including nurse practitioners and medical doctors all with their corresponding licensures. It sounded like such an awesome thing. They offered a larger variety of services for the patients, a killer business model, and all the while, they were very profitable each month. I thought this should be my endgame. When we started GSW, 1 made sure our name didn't have the word "chiropractic" in it, to leave that door open for the future, a possible integration.

I imagined that I would be a chiropractor and the owner of an entity that has multiple specialties working together for the collective good of the patient (and for generating revenue).

Over time, I've heard of many horror stories of how several of these medically integrated chiropractic offices ended up shutting the medical portion and returning to their chiropractic roots. Medical integration can often be a large hassle due to the overhead that comes with paying for the licensure and the additional liability. This additional overhead expenditure and added risk exposure leads to a lot of stress.

In our practice, we run a higher overhead in comparison to a small chiropractic clinic. However, our services and our additional revenue is being generated under the scope of a chiropractic license. The philosophy all jives with a natural healthcare approach. We don't have to bring in highly paid healthcare practitioners like nurses and medical doctors. Not to say that's always a bad thing. I'm just sharing how this concept of departmentalizing works the way it does at GSW.

You can departmentalize your clinic and have different departments that generate additional services and revenue for the clinic. In addition to our exercise department, we also have a traction department and an X-ray suite. These are all various departments within one clinic. Having specific roles for staff that can add more valuable services for your patients generates additional revenue and adds to that bottom line every single month, which is super helpful.

The key to running successful departments within your clinic is pairing the right staff member with the role that is best suited to play to their strengths and their specific skills. For example, with Tony's background in the fitness arena and his natural ability to come up with ideas for improved procedures and solutions, he has been an excellent addition to our fitness area.

If you're reading this book, it probably means that you are at a different level as compared to the average chiropractor. Likely, you want to learn the ways that others are successfully implementing these procedures and protocols on a larger scale.

My goal in sharing all of this is to save you time and energy and prevent you from having to make frustrating and costly mistakes. A bigger goal of mine is to build a trusted relationship with you. As you implement the things that we share in this book, this will bring you closer to a higher level of clinical excellence. This will help accomplish my ultimate goal, which is to elevate the quality and the image of our profession by building and gathering a network of chiropractors that share in this vision.

When a patient walks into your office and understands your unique approach, they should be blown away and feel as though that they are in the right place. We have had patients who had nearly given up on chiropractic care until they came to see us. On a patient's initial visit, they will oftentimes tell us how radically different our approach is compared to the last chiropractor they saw. So the time is now. Let's set a new precedence for our profession! And on that high note, now we will cover a topic that makes me tired just thinking about it, but we have to cover it. That is none other than a word that rhymes with "thrilling": billing.

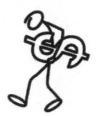

CHAPTER 16

Billing

I AM NOT GOING TO BORE YOU WITH THE MECHANICS OF billing but, rather, what works for us at GSW. I do break this down in more detail in our MoveWell University program.

First and foremost, when it comes to billing, pay attention to different rules in your state. They can play a large role in the decisions you make as far as what services you can provide, in addition to being well-educated on how health insurance really works. I recently heard from a doctor who is doing well in practice and wanted to know if this program would be right for her. When discussing an exercise department, she mentioned she doesn't work with insurance at all and she felt as if she would have to start to accept health insurance in order to incorporate an exercise department into her practice. That is not the case. You do not have to go through insurance to do exercise!

Some states and some doctors I've worked with say, "If you're in network with XYZ insurance, they cover a maximum of $60 per visit for anything and everything that you do." And of course, "You can't bill the patient for the difference." Sure, if that's the case. It's a crummy contract to have. I would recommend to find out what it would take to get out of network with that particular carrier. For instance, it may be a different story if your exercise department is a completely separate business with a different tax ID number. If that is the case, you may not be subject to these same rules that are spelled out in the insurance contract. This would be a great question for your attorney.

Approximately one-third of our patients are self-pay (do not have or elect to use their health insurance). With insurance companies having expensive deductibles, offering a self-pay option is important, as it can be more affordable for the patient. The self-pay option can also be an automatic monthly debited payment, which many of our patients prefer. For further financial options, we utilize ChiroHealthUSA. This provides patients with the opportunity to pay for their care and get the savings benefits with a compliant fee schedule system. We talk about this in detail in our program, or if you want to know more, you can talk to ChiroHealthUSA.

At GSW, we work with private health insurance companies, personal injury cases, and a little bit or worker's compensation. We have several objective measures to identify the necessity for care. Then the services are carefully documented, and we make sure we pay attention to which codes are time-specific and recognize the other little nuances that makes the billing aspect so intimidating (and frustrating). The good news is once you learn the rules, you just make sure you play by those rules, and you usually will not have a problem. In my experience, most of the stories that I hear about how chiropractors are having problems with getting paid by personal health insurance usually involve extremely sub-par documentation. If the notes are not up to speed, forget about it. You won't win. You have to decide if it's worth the time and energy to ensure that you are documenting properly. I would say it's a no-brainer. Insurance billing aside, thorough documentation is for your protection. So get to it!

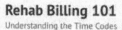

Rehab Billing 101
Understanding the Time Codes

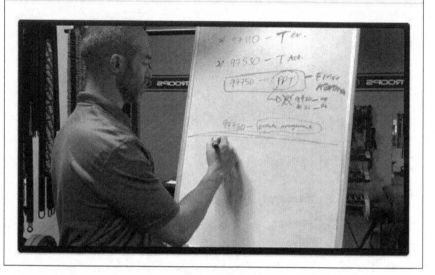

Understanding the rules regarding time specific procedures is crucial to make sure you are billing in an appropriate fashion.

Aside from appropriate documentation in our SOAP notes, we stay organized by utilizing our travel card (covered in a previous chapter) that goes with the patient throughout the clinic during each visit. As we provide multiple services that day, it keeps everything organized. We use a recommendation card to organize and plan out a patient's care. It allows for the doctor to clearly identify the clinical protocols, home care, and duration of care. The completed card is then given to our billing department. The billing staff can then design a financial plan that is accurate and best meets the needs of the patient. We currently use the Cash Plan Calculator in Cash Practice, which as the name implies, allows us to factor in self-pay plans for the patient. Additionally, it is designed to calculate the patient portion when utilizing health insurance. It will assist in factoring in deductibles, co-pays, co-insurances, and non-covered services.

In addition, it's important that ALL of our staff understands the billing aspects to some degree, not just the billing department. If everyone has some clarity into how billing works, it's helpful when decisions need to be made last minute or if a staff member is asked by a patient, "Why did I only get six visits?" The staff can very likely help field that question while it is fresh and explain where the patient is with their care. With everyone on the same page, the patient won't receive conflicting information.

If you want more information about billing, I suggest that you check your insurance contracts. You can also talk to Chiro-HealthUSA and let them know that we sent you (and they'll take extra-special care of you). When you become part of MoveWell University, we share our forms for setting up our fee schedule with ChiroHealthUSA and we go through this in more detail.

In the next chapter, let's cover the launch.

CHAPTER 17

Launching MoveWell

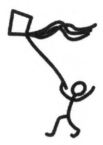

O NCE YOU HAVE FOLLOWED ALL OF THE STEPS AND parameters we've given you in "MoveWell Secrets," start preparing for takeoff! Understand that it's not going to be perfect and it will be a bit stressful. It will require 110 percent from you, but you can and will be successful! Don't wait for the "perfect moment." It doesn't exist. Immerse yourself in preparing and enjoy the process.

When I started implementing Chiropractic BioPhysics in my practice in New Mexico, it really became the foundation for Move-Well. I just didn't know it at the time. It's where I immersed myself in learning everything I could. I wanted my patients and the community to know about the amazing stuff I was learning. I would discuss this new information with my patients during adjustments to get the word out about this new exciting addition to my practice. Plus, they could see how excited I was!

I taught weekly workshops to my patients. In the 60 minutes I had allotted, I wanted my patients and the community to know about this revolutionary new approach I was learning that could take their health and function to an entirely new level.

So where do you start? How do you begin launching MoveWell into your practice?

Begin by setting goals. Being goal-oriented is something we really focus on at GSW. As you begin setting goals for your own business, share these goals with your team so everyone can share in the same vision. Talk with your team with excitement and enthusiasm for new opportunities! If they see you're excited, they'll stand with you. As you're setting goals, don't do what I did and spend month after month with three to four hours of sleep each night.

Here's my shameless plug — totally shameless!

Do you know why I feel NO SHAME? Because I know how much it took for us to create all of these shortcuts. I know how much time and energy this will save you. So do yourself a HUGE favor. Launch corrective exercise into your practice with the help of MoveWell University. This is a no-brainer.

Like I said, the majority of work that had to be created and tried and tested has already been done. We have the bases covered for you, so you can get more sleep than I did. As you go through the sections in MoveWell University, make notes because you have a lot of work ahead of you!

Now, back to the goal-setting.

As you are setting goals and planning, what needs to be dealt with first? Is it physical space? Exercise equipment? If you're looking into expanding your physical space, attention to detail must be given to planning. If you will need to change the architecture of your clinic, knock a wall down, or conduct a more minor remodel, make sure to future-pace the process. Map out how many patients can be seen at one time in the space, and before you launch this with your patients, have your staff go through the process. Can you expand into the space in phases, or do you need to jump in and take over all of the space at once? As far as goals, put a date on a calendar and commit to it. That is the first day that your very first patient will begin this program. You have to get started somewhere.

You may feel you have to wait to implement until you've mastered everything. It's quite the contrary. Just go! Jump! Get to it!

Once you have the foundation down, you understand the components covered in this book, and if you have taken my advice and used our systems in MoveWell University to accelerate this process, then you have to trust the system. Go through all of the modules inside of the MWU membership site at least once. Then begin. Continue to refine and study the material, let it further sink in, discover the questions that you will inevitably ask once the process is in motion, and then turn to the resources within MWU. You will not be able to be fully prepared for everything. Get the basics down: mobility first, then stability. Understand the basic flexibility exercises for hip mobility and thoracic mobility; those are the two most common issues that you'll find within the patient population. Get familiar with how to explain WHY your patients need to be doing this, and then again, just jump in.

Then ask yourself this question: What do you want for your practice?

If you want to implement all the components of MoveWell University, then great! Or do you want to only utilize certain aspects. It's not an all-or-nothing thing. I tend to err on the side of giving people too much and that's Ok. (We do think we have the best system ever for this type of setup).

When we first began to organize GSW, we started with a personal trainer who was going to run the fitness department (similar to an independent contractor). She was great with her clients and had great knowledge in personal training. But it wasn't what we wanted for our patients, and this trainer had a different set of views. Needless to say, it does take time to hire the right staff, and it seems like we'd find one great person for every three people we'd hire. Once you find them, keep them! They will be the hardworking people who help further develop the systems along the way and will have an obvious excitement about what they are doing. It is now to the point where training is very efficient at GSW, as we now use the same Move-Well University membership site that you will have access to. That's our main vehicle for our staff training. I spent months putting these protocols together, and I am confident that my staff is well-trained. Yours can be too!

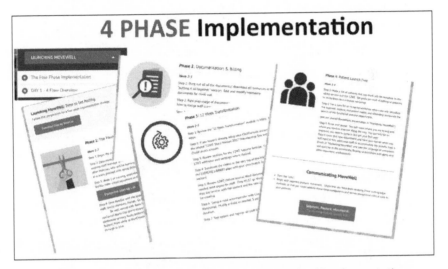

The MoveWell University program has an organized implementation process to help make sure these systems are launched successfully. (www.MoveWellUniversity.com)

Hire before you begin! Just like a restaurant planning their grand opening, they hire their staff and spend anywhere between two and six weeks training before they open the doors. You don't want your new staff to become overwhelmed and burned out. Things are going to change rapidly, so be ahead of the game. Typically, depending on the skillset of one of our exercise staff, we expect that they can handle a weekly patient load of approximately 40 to 60 visits on their own. But make sure they are spaced out, and don't forget compliance rules with certain insurance contracts! As things pick up, which they will quickly. Hire three to four weeks in advance of the predicted growth, to allow time for the new staff member to properly train on the MoveWell University membership site. Look at your trends and by hiring early. You have time for new staff to shadow under your experienced therapists.

Once you have two staff members, you'll soon expand to three. Before you know it, your exercise area is able to handle well over 150 visits per week. In our practice, we also have some backup staff, so in times of heavy volume, there is help!

Communicate with your staff frequently! Every week our team has meetings. We address what needs to be talked about for as long as needed (plan for 90 minutes). In addition, we have with small group meetings during the week to keep everyone on the same page. Do not lose the component of communication. No matter where you are in implementing changes at your business, communication with staff must remain continuously available.

Since you cannot do this without a team, always include them in discussions. Inclusion is appreciated. For example, in the inter-actions I have with my exercise staff, I'm asking them what is going smoothly and what are some hurdles they are experiencing. I ask for their ideas on how to improve any of these areas that seem to be throwing them a curveball.

Tony liked this approach, stating: "I really appreciate whenever Dr. Todd's proposing some kind of change to the exercise depart-ment. Dr. Todd asks us what we think, and we discuss changes to make them as effective as possible. It gives everyone a chance to bounce ideas around, which is how we initially prepared for the 12-Week Transformation before that launched back in late 2016. During a group meeting, Dr. Todd announced what we were doing for the New Year and we would all go through the modules of the 12-Week Transformation as a team. And we all did it!"

Another important component to weekly staff training and constant communication is learning the objections patients tell the staff but they don't ever tell you. Many times, the exercise staff will spend so much time with the patient, they end up hearing objections patients may have about their care (or awesome feedback). You want your staff to understand the value of the care that your patient is receiving. If there's an objection verbalized regarding certain exercises or a patient is expressing, they are going to drop out of care. Your staff needs to be able to identify the objection and address it. The timing on these situations can be a game-changer, and a motivated, excited, and well-trained member of your team is crucial for resolving these events.

I suggest practicing running through objections with your staff members before you launch your functional movement exercise department. We created some video scenarios for handing patient objections with effective communication skills. For instance, objections can vary from "Can I just do this at home?" or "I can't afford to do this" to "I just did my exercises before I came in, so I don't have to do them here in the office and shouldn't have to pay for them." You want your exercise staff (and all staff for that matter) to be able to respond to these statements without hesitation.

Next, this is not a sprint. It's a marathon, so pace yourself!

When you start off and need equipment (yet aren't ready to buy everything), start with less equipment. Do a prediction of how many patients you have right now and the patient visits per week that you are currently doing and what you think that will go up to. Typically, if you're doing a promotion in office, you can very likely get 30 to 40 percent of your active patients to engage in the activity. This is great, as you can invite your patients to include their family, friends, co-workers, etc. in the promotion. You're doing something great for your existing patients, while providing valuable education to potential patients. Don't forget your old patients! Give them a reason to resume their care if they have gone missing in action. By reaching out to them and letting them know you're doing new, you can use this as a reactivation campaign. Offering a complimentary movement assessment can be used. But be careful. You don't want to devalue your services.

Before you launch with "live" patients, have your staff train and practice with family and friends. Provide the opportunity to go through everything and catch any mistakes. When you launch with patients, you need to be ok with the fact that everything is not going to be perfect, but like the saying goes, "Better done than perfect." When you make mistakes (and you will make mistakes), try to make most of those with your staff and friends.

Trust me, if there had been a program out there that offered a smooth step-by-step process for me to implement this exercise department into my clinic — where the kinks were worked out — I would have paid for it. When I originally launched this myself, I spent a lot of money to fly experts out to us to do weekend trainings. I feel like I spent every waking moment of my life creating and modifying forms and writing up procedure ideas. Then I would turn around and completely reinvent the process again and again, until we got it right. With so much information out there, it became important to figure out what works clinically and then organize it in such a way to work efficiently with our daily patient flow in our clinic.

In the end, the launch of a corrective exercise and functional movement department is a huge resource and service that you will be offering your community. This will enable you to better serve your patients and help them improve their lives in a major way. Go you!

CHAPTER 18

Marketing MoveWell

R EMEMBER HOW MOVEWELL UNIVERSITY BEGAN. THIS was originally a program that we designed for fitness professionals, not chiropractors. Then, about a month or so into designing it, we realized this needed to be a chiropractic program, and we changed our direction. With that change of pace, we still wanted to eventually come back around and complete the program that was initially intended for the fitness professional community. We did that. Now we have a full-blown automated marketing arm of MoveWell University that enables all of the members of MWU to go out and develop relationships with the fitness professionals and personal trainers in their community. This is called MoveWell University for Fitness Professionals, and it's awesome. I'll cover that in a minute.

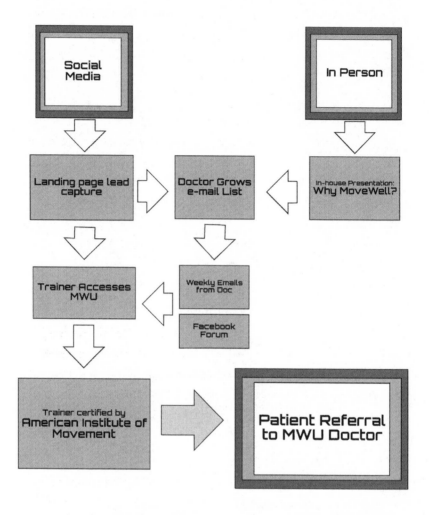

Marketing MoveWell is an automated program for fitness professionals. This flow chart illustrates the big picture and how all of these
steps work in order to make this successful.

Let me first share the background of how I used to connect with
personal trainers. Before there was MoveWell University for Fitness
Professionals, we went to gyms and we would teach a 90-minute
seminar about functional movement to their trainers. We would do
this in multiple modules, which is a time commitment and time
investment, but it is invaluable and it works well. That's where the

MoveWell University for Fitness Professionals helps share this knowledge even further. The personal trainers can access the information on their own time, which is often preferred. Plus, with a certification that we put in place, they're motivated to go through the program.

So now that we touched on MWU-Fitness Professionals, the next step in implementing this exercise department is marketing to the community. This is vital for your business to succeed. One of the main reasons we incorporated corrective exercise and functional movement in our facility was so we could reach more people and get the message out there and differentiate ourselves in the community. When marketing functional movement to personal trainers, gyms are an obvious starting point.

CrossFit gyms are great to start with, as their trainers are required to have some level of functional movement understanding. Many "big box" gyms have recently incorporated more functional training as well, because they're realizing the isolated machine training is becoming a thing of the past. Exhaust all of the fitness and exercise places first. Within the Marketing MoveWell module inside of the "Pro" section of MoveWell University, we cover how to approach the gyms and the most effective methods that we have tried and tested to develop referral relationships with personal trainers.

As you become more comfortable with the process of reaching out to personal trainers, you can expand out into gymnastics, for example. Functional movement is this universal language that brings you into all kinds of places that you would have likely never been able to get into. Once you start thinking about wellness in this way, all of a sudden, you will see all of these possibilities open.

MoveWell University for Fitness Professionals is a different version compared to the MoveWell University that is designed for chiropractors. A portion of the content crosses over, but one of the biggest differences and attractions for the personal trainer is they can achieve a certification by the credentialing agency for MWU-Fitness Professionals, The American Institute of Movement. This process is fully automated, the trainers have an online test that they will need to complete to show they can demonstrate competency in the subject matter, and when they pass, they will be able to print out a customized certificate with their name on it.

When marketing to fitness professionals, you're giving them an easy action step for referring someone to you who has hit a stopping point in their exercise program or is suffering from an injury. Your job is to teach the fitness professional how to make these judgment calls and not be afraid of losing the client. On the contrary, you will help prevent the client from quitting their training and likely never returning. You're reassuring them it's a team effort to get their client back to them. That's one of the processes that we've automated inside of Marketing MoveWell.

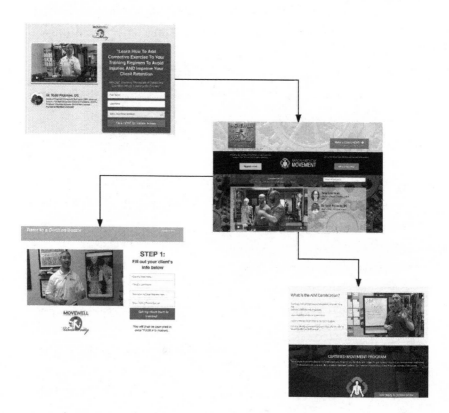

Fitness professionals can easily fill out the client's information and send the referral your way. You can further build these relationships by reaching out to the trainer and thanking them for the referral, and, with the patient's permission, fill them in on the clinical findings with their client. This creates great relationships that have the ultimate goal of helping someone get better. Create a goal together to get these patients back on track and healthy!

One of the main reasons that I was initially inspired to develop our exercise department (besides the obvious improvement in patient results) was because I knew it was going to open so many other platforms for other practitioners and fitness professionals. And it has done that. With the current state of health in this country, and so many Americans being overweight, the fitness and movement topic is a hot one. Even if they aren't doing it, the community acknowledges the importance of fitness. YOU need to connect the dots for them. You show them they are missing a huge piece of the picture.

If they are jumping into an exercise program without a proper assessment, they are likely making the mistake that Gray Cook calls "stacking fitness on top of dysfunction," which is a recipe for painful injuries and even longer recoveries. You may also find many of your patients understand the value of movement but have had a bad experience with exercise. You and your staff need to be able to connect with them in a unique way that might light a spark inside them that they so badly need.

What about marketing in the community to medical clinics?

This has been huge for us! Some weeks, we go to one or two clinics and talk with healthcare practitioners and show them a variety of the comparative, objective results that we collect to substantiate our care. We highlight the corrective exercise and functional movement, and we show them pictures of the facility and how this works and how people are improving. They love it.

Medical doctors are used to referring their patients to physical therapists. That is what they are comfortable with. When they see how it's "like" physical therapy, it's as if a light bulb goes on and they feel more comfortable referring a patient to a chiropractor. This is different from what they are used to when they imagine a chiropractic approach.

This has continued to be one of our biggest sources for new patient referrals. Medical clinics have been referring to us left and right. Healthcare practitioners are realizing ours is a specialized clinic and we do things different.

Now let's cover the last part of this chapter and this book, a few more aspects of staff training.

I'm excited about the MoveWell University program because we are pioneers in this space. It's never been done before, and I'm watching other chiropractors around the country implement these systems and quickly and successfully meet their goals and projections. This program is a fit for a lot of chiropractors who might be intimidated to do something new. If you're already this far and you're engaged in this material, save yourself some time, energy, and money and don't try to invent it all on your own. It's already done and ready to go!

In closing, I appreciate you spending the time to read this book and hang out with me. If you haven't already, I encourage you to go online and sign up for one of our FREE online webinars where we go into more detail about the MoveWell University program. If you're ready to jump in, you can get instant access, unlock all the modules inside MoveWell University, and start implementing this into your practice. If you're planning on this for the future, I hope this book has helped you feel more prepared.

MoveWell and prosper.

— Todd Pickman, DC

JOIN OUR GROUP OF DOCTORS THAT ARE USING MOVEWELL UNIVERSITY TO DIAL IN THEIR EXERCISE DEPARTMENT:
WWW.MOVEWELLUNIVERSITY.COM